STATE INTERVENTION
IN MEDICAL CARE

STATE INTERVENTION IN MEDICAL CARE

Consequences for Britain, France, Sweden, and the United States, 1890–1970

J. ROGERS HOLLINGSWORTH
JERALD HAGE
ROBERT A. HANNEMAN

CORNELL UNIVERSITY PRESS

Ithaca and London

First published 1990 by Cornell University Press

International Standard Book Number 0-8014-2389-9 (cloth)
International Standard Book Number 0-8014-9615-2 (paper)
Library of Congress Catalog Card Number 89-25155

Printed in the United States of America

Librarians: Library of Congress cataloging information appears on the last page of the book.

⊗ The paper used in this publication meets the minimum requirements of the American National Standard for Permanence of Paper for Printed Library Materials Z39.48—1984.

For Ellen Jane,
Madeleine, and Pat

CONTENTS

ACKNOWLEDGMENTS

This project began when all three of us were at the University of Wisconsin. In a stimulating interdisciplinary environment, we decided to combine the study of public policy and institutional change, using historical and cross-national analysis. In several publications we have attempted to understand why various institutional arrangements emerge and why specific types of consequences result from variation in institutional forms. This book addresses the latter issue: How has variation in institutional forms influenced the performance of the medical systems of Great Britain, France, Sweden, and the United States since 1890?

In writing this book, we have deliberately attempted to combine several areas of scholarship: organizational theory, political science, and political sociology with their concerns with power and conflict; medical sociology; and macrohistorical analysis. A remarkable number of friends and colleagues have commented on various parts of the study, including Jens Alber, Odin Anderson, Gerhard Lehmbruch, Renate Mayntz, Tom McCraw, Ron Numbers, Fritz Scharpf, Burt Weisbrod, and Erik O. Wright. Many others have shared their ideas about various aspects of the project. Alfred Chandler and Oliver Williamson have taught us much about the emergence of specific types of institutional arrangements, and from Robert Fogel we have learned about the problems of measuring health with historical materials. At a critical juncture in the project, Ellen Jane Hollingsworth read the entire manuscript and helped shape its structure. Her assistance has been invaluable. In addition, our colleagues in the History of Medicine and in the Sociology of Medicine at the University of Wisconsin have on separate occasions invited us to share our ideas with them; these experiences were very helpful in clarifying our ideas.

Over time, many people have provided enormous assistance in collecting and analyzing data for various tables. They include Andy Aoki, Dan Bailey, Fred Burkhard, Ralph Coates, Jody Davis, Margaret Hedstrom, Steve Johnson, Kelly Joyce, Lisa MacPherson, Frank Monfort, George Pasdirtz, and Stuart Rossmiller.

John Klingenstein and the Esther A. and Joseph Klingenstein Fund, Inc., of New York City have supported the work of the senior author on several projects. Their confidence and generosity is much appreciated. Financial support for this and related projects was also provided by the National Science Foundation under grant SOC 76-17318; the German Marshall Fund of the United States; the Graduate Research Committee and the Institute for Research on Poverty of the University of Wisconsin; the Rockefeller Foundation Study and Conference Center in Bellagio, Italy; and the Woodrow Wilson International Center for Scholars.

In addition, we express our gratitude to Professor John Simon of Yale University. Using his good offices to provide funding for various research projects, he has over the years been a special benefactor for the senior author by facilitating grants from Yale University's Program in Law, Science, and Medicine and the Program on Non-Profit Organizations. His exceptional collegiality and willingness to invest enormous energy to assist the research of others are appreciated far beyond our ability to express here.

We especially thank Sandy Heitzkey, Jane Mesler, Anita Olson, and Paula Pfannes for the typing of many drafts of the manuscript, always in a cheerful and efficient manner.

Finally, we express our appreciation to our wives, who have made many sacrifices over the years so that we might work together on this project. As a token of our love and appreciation, we dedicate this book to them.

J. ROGERS HOLLINGSWORTH
JERALD HAGE
ROBERT A. HANNEMAN

STATE INTERVENTION
IN MEDICAL CARE

1

THEORETICAL PERSPECTIVES: AN INTRODUCTION

For some years, there has been growing concern in Western Europe and the United States about the effectiveness of medical delivery systems. In most nations costs have risen rapidly, while mortality and other measures of population health have improved only slowly. Enormous gains have been made in medical technology, yet in many nations some social classes continue to suffer poor health and have limited access to high quality services. Increasingly, matters of medical policy have become part of the national political agenda, often provoking bitter debate among providers, state officials, and various groups of consumers.

At the core of the debate about the effectiveness of medical technology and the efficiency of medical systems is the question of state intervention: how large a role should the state play in regulating and providing services? Proponents of "privatization" argue that the more the state intervenes in the delivery of medical care, the more inefficient the system becomes; others want an increased governmental role. In the United States the demand for a national health service is once again on the political agenda. For either viewpoint, proponents can bring to bear well-articulated theories of why state intervention ought to improve (or worsen) the performance of medical systems, and yet there has been surprisingly little empirical research on the consequences of state intervention or privatization in the delivery of medical services for an entire nation.

It is particularly appropriate to examine the effects of state intervention and privatization on the performance of medical delivery systems
now, at a time of renewed interest in the study of the state within the
social sciences. The list of important studies seeking to explain the
emergence of the "active state" (Orloff and Skocpol, 1984; Tilly, 1975;
Skocpol, 1981; Carnoy, 1984; Evans, Rueschemeyer, and Skocpol,
1985; Alford and Friedland, 1985) is expanding. The focus of most
such work, however, has been state building, the changing role of the
state in a capitalist society, or the role of state officials in the development of particular policies or the passage of specific legislation. This
literature does not extensively address how state intervention affects
the way systems perform.

During the 1970s, several comparative studies of national medical
systems were published (Abel-Smith, 1976; Marmor and Thomas,
1971; Andersen, Smedby, and Anderson, 1970; Anderson, 1972;
Glaser, 1970). Usually these focused on institutional differences, such
as the number of hospital beds per capita, payment procedures, visits
to the doctor per capita, and performance measures such as mortality
rates and costs (Hollingsworth, 1986). As a result, we now know a great
deal about the medical systems of other countries, but their differences
have not been systematically related to variations in the way they are
organized.

This book attempts to speak to these and other questions about the
impact of state intervention on the performance of medical delivery
systems in Western Europe and North America. Specifically, it explores
how changes in the degree of state intervention influence system performance. Its format is a cross-national, historical comparison of the
medical systems of Great Britain, France, Sweden, and the United
States during the period between 1890–1970.

We have chosen these four countries because they have differed
greatly in degree of state intervention and privatization during the past
century. All four societies have experienced substantial increases in
state activity, but in considerably different ways. The varied levels and
rates of change in state activity provide an ideal opportunity for testing
hypotheses about how state intervention influences delivery system performance.

The impact of changes in state intervention on the behavior of medical delivery systems must be understood in the context of other
changes that have occurred in these four countries—changes both specific to their medical delivery systems and more generally to their societies and economies. Hence, we will be concerned in the following
chapters with the interaction of changes in the role of the state with

changes in human capital and medical technology and with other socio-economic changes in the larger society.

The vast increase in medical knowledge during the past century has been increasingly embodied in both human and physical capital. The years 1890 and 1970 nicely bracket the emergence of the "modern" hospital as a critical arena for medical care, the rise of complexity in medical technology, and the increase in the number of physicians (Hollingsworth and Hollingsworth, 1987; Hollingsworth, 1986). These changes, in turn, have tended to encourage state intervention to finance, coordinate, and provide access to changing medical technology.

In assessing the impact of privatization and state intervention on the way medical systems perform, we must be careful to take into consideration how changes in human capital also shape the performance of medical systems. Do medical systems behave as they do because they are privatized or state controlled or is much of their behavior shaped by the increased investment in human capital and changes in specialized technology?

Denison's classic works on education and its impact on productivity and growth (1962, 1967, 1974) have generated a great deal of interest in human capital. As yet, there has been little research on the relationship between investment in medical education and such measures of performance as mortality, costs, and efficiency (see the discussion in Schneyer, Landefield, and Sandifer, 1981). In the medical area the level of human capital investment has increased in two major ways. First, the number of physicians (and other medical personnel) per capita has grown, and second, the levels of skill, knowledge, and training of medical practitioners have improved. Unquestionably, such changes in human capital directly affect the performance of medical delivery systems, regardless of the form and extent of state intervention. They also influence the nature of state intervention and thus indirectly affect system performance by modifying the role the state plays in coordinating the delivery of medical services. By conceptualizing the problem in this way, we can better understand how investment in human capital, changes in medical technology, and the nature of state intervention are interrelated.

Other societal forces must also be considered. France, Great Britain, Sweden, and the United States vary in population size, density, and ethnocultural homogeneity; level of economic development; institutional history; and timing of industrialization and modernization. Clearly, changes in system performance, state intervention, investment in human capital, and medical technology are grounded in these societal contexts, and we must be sensitive to their influence.

New Directions in Institutional Analysis

The recent interest in the state is part of a resurgence of institutional analysis in the social sciences (see Meyer and Rowan; 1977; Meyer and Scott, 1983; DiMaggio and Powell, 1983; Hollingsworth, 1986; Zucker, 1987; Scott, 1987; Weisbrod, 1988; Williamson, 1975, 1985; North, 1981; Streeck and Schmitter, 1985; Schmitter, 1977; and Katzenstein, 1984). Much of this literature explores why certain institutional arrangements emerge, why market, corporatist, or state institutional forms of coordination come into being. In this investigation, historical research has proved to be a key tool for scholars interested not only in why institutions emerge but also in which specific policies countries adopt. For example, in order to explain why one form of national health insurance or social security emerged rather than another, many institutionalists have turned to detailed historical case studies (Skocpol and Ikenberry, 1983; Skocpol and Amenta, 1986; Orloff and Skocpol, 1984).

Some of the most interesting institutionalist perspectives have demonstrated how the institutional environment of organizations shapes the kinds of institutions which emerge (Meyer and Scott, 1983). Nevertheless, we know too little about the *actual behavior* of institutions; we must ask to what extent the actual behavior of institutions is consistent with the myths societies hold about it. Do institutions have reputations for behaving one way when in fact their behavior is entirely the opposite? In confronting this key problem, this book departs from the type of institutional analysis previously done. Rather than try to explain why different institutional arrangements emerge or why one type of policy rather than another is chosen, we want to consider what consequences follow from specific types of institutional forms, to see if popular beliefs about the behavior of institutions diverge from actual behavior. For example, many in Europe and the United States believe that the marketplace is the most efficient coordinator of economic activity; others believe that state intervention is best for achieving social equality. In this book we want to study the relevance of these assertions for medical systems. By outlining the consequences of specific institutional arrangements on key performances, we hope to discover if it is possible that one institutional form might maximize both efficiency and egalitarian goals.

As long as such assertions are unchallenged by scholarly analysis, particular institutional arrangements may remain in force, achieving goals just the opposite of what societies intend. Indeed, elites in both public and private organizations often believe they are accomplishing certain objectives, when in fact they are not, and in most countries there are deeply ingrained myths about the efficaciousness of state and privatized institutional forms (Meyer and Scott, 1983).

Much of the recent debate about medical care in Europe and the United States has been over what consequences follow from a privatized or state form of coordination. This book assumes that what works best in one sector of the economy does not necessarily work best in another—that different institutional forms have different consequences across industries. Thus, we hope to shed some light on what is different about medical care and why the consequences of privatization or state coordination in the medical area might be different from the consequences of similar policies in manufacturing or other sectors. One goal of our work is to begin constructing a theory about the logics involved in different institutional forms in varying economic sectors and different societies—in this instance the logics of privatized and state forms of coordination in the delivery of medical care. In one sense, our work is relevant to the current interest of many social scientists in the logic of markets and hierarchies (Williamson, 1975, 1985). Whereas they have explored why certain institutional forms emerge, we propose to specify the logics or social processes that connect certain institutional arrangements with various kinds of performance.

Unquestionably, understanding why specific institutional forms emerge when they do is an intellectual issue of profound importance, but we do not raise this issue here. Instead, we want to set a new agenda in institutional analysis. We want to understand the consequences of different institutional forms in terms of efficiency, better health, lower costs, innovation, and equality. By focusing institutional analysis in this way, we hope to make it highly relevant to the current public policy debates in Europe and North America.

New Directions in Policy Analysis

Most Western societies wish to have innovative medical technologies, healthier populations, socially efficient medical care, and egalitarian, low-cost medical systems. The policy literature, however, has not been very helpful in suggesting institutional arrangements that optimize these goals. Moreover, these goals often conflict with one another. The highly egalitarian system may also be highly standardized and not very innovative; the highly innovative system may not be socially efficient.

Policy making about medical systems is usually highly specific and incremental. Countries, like organizations, are less likely to engage in comprehensive strategic planning than to react to specific problems

with piecemeal policy (Mintzberg, 1979; Lindblom, 1959). For example, in recent years, the American government has adopted a multi-
plicity of policies to contain the costs of medical care. The past two
decades have seen certificate-of-need legislation, the introduction of
Professional Standard Review Organizations and health maintenance
organizations, and attempts to contain rises in hospital costs for Medicare patients. These policies, however, have not been very successful.
Certain underlying institutional arrangements in the American medical
system strongly influence the level of medical expenditures, and individual policies that do not alter the basic institutional arrangement of
the delivery system are not likely to have much influence in slowing the
rate of increase in medical expenditures (Hollingsworth, 1986).

Our approach to the analysis of medical policy emphasizes the importance of these larger institutional and structural constraints on the
performance of national medical delivery systems, rather than the evaluation of particular pieces of legislation. Even within this broader
focus, however, the role of the state is critical: the state is one of the
few institutions with sufficient power to alter the large-scale structural
patterns that account for most of the variability in the performance of
national medical systems.

Perhaps the central importance of state intervention in the delivery
of medical services can be better appreciated if we understand why it
has not been a focus of research, even though it lies at the heart of the
current debate over privatization. Why should obvious questions about
the social impact of state intervention be missed both in the policy literature and in most academic research? The answer is complex but in
part lies in the dominance of neoclassical microeconomic theory as the
central paradigm in policy analysis at the level of the nation-state. In
the medical area (and in a number of others), however, the laws of
supply and demand—especially at the nation-state level—do not operate as neoclassical economic theory predicts.

The tendency to analyze the behavior of medical systems through the
laws of the marketplace has led to an emphasis on micro-level studies
of physicians and hospitals rather than macro-level studies of organizational systems and the state. Indeed, neoclassical economic theory tends
to see the state as an afterthought (if at all), not as an active agent that
transforms and shapes "supply," "demand," "prices," and even "economic rationality." If the consequences of state intervention are to be
understood in the medical area, state mechanisms should not be reduced to the management of "market imperfection" and "market failure." The valuable insights of neoclassical economic theory need to be
augmented by an expanded perspective that includes nonmarket mechanisms, especially the state. If we are to understand why medical sys-

tems perform as they do, we must add to the ideas of supply and demand the concepts of planning, programming, and control. One of the
major objectives of this book is to advance the theory of the state by
beginning to explicate how state mechanisms of coordination and control operate.

Our position is that there is a need for policy analyses of alternative
institutional arrangements in social services which recognize two essential facts: (1) privatization is a more appropriate concept for understanding social services than markets, and (2) state hierarchies are an
important alternative to privatization. Our objective is to begin the development of an institutional theory relative to privatization and state
hierarchies. While there are several literatures that are germane, they
generally do not focus on the social consequences of alternative institutional arrangements. For example, transaction-cost economics attempts
to explain the emergence and persistence of markets or corporate hierarchies as institutional forms, but it does not systematically consider the
consequences of an institutional form.

Similarly, the theory of markets is not exactly relevant, since much of
the discussion in the area of social services—and medical care in particular—focuses on privatization, which involves a broader perspective
than the theory of markets. Privatization involves both market and
nonmarket activity in the private sector (Starr, 1985). The concept of
privatization is more appropriate for the study of medical care since
the state has long restricted the extent of market activity by licensing
physicians and hospitals and by establishing standards for hospitals and
medical education.

At the same time, the logic underlying the arguments of proponents
of privatization is very much about markets: namely, physicians and
hospitals in the private sector will be more efficient if they can compete
with one another than will be the case under a system in which physicians are employed and hospitals are owned by the state (Manga and
Weller, 1980; Weller and Manga, 1983; Hollingsworth, 1986). Even
though there has been a great deal of ideological discussion about the
effects of privatization, the subject has not been studied at the level of
the nation-state, which is nevertheless the most appropriate level for
comparing the social performances of hierarchies and privatization in
the medical sector.

This study differs from most policy studies in several respects. One
type of policy study, usually in political science or sociology, focuses on
how a particular policy was determined by structural and institutional
factors and the relative power of specific interest groups. Whether the
decision is to adopt a national health insurance program, to employ all
the doctors in the public sector, to provide kidney dialysis at public

expense to all who need it—the conventional approach tends to concentrate on the arena of battle, the strategy and tactics of the relevant interest groups engaged in the political struggle to adopt some particular legislation. What is usually missing is an analysis of the consequences of a particular policy. This lack is somewhat surprising, for what is at stake in such political struggles is the outcome foreseen by the combatants. At issue is what effect a given political action will have on system performance. Our research concentrates not on causes but on consequences of large-scale institutional changes (particularly changes in types of state intervention) on system performance.

Another important and valuable tradition in policy analysis is program evaluation. Cost-benefit studies of particular treatments or payment systems are especially numerous in the medical policy literature, for example. Most such studies focus on the microlevel, however, and although informative, they do not address a whole range of questions relative to the organization of national medical systems. We maintain that the behavior or performance of entire medical systems is far more than the sum of the performance of its parts.

We contend that the behavior of national medical systems is very much influenced by variations in forms of state intervention and privatization, investment in human capital, the level of system complexity, and the societal context in which the system is located. Those who want to maximize such goals as cost-effectiveness, equality of access, innovativeness, and better health must recognize that simple tinkering with the system by means of a new piece of legislation here and there is not likely to have marked effects on performance. Institutional performance can, however, be modified by structural changes, and the state is central to any attempt to restructure Western medical systems.

Most of the debate about privatization in the neoclassical literature about markets and the state has dealt primarily with the issue of efficiency or waste. We propose to broaden the paradigm, first, by carefully conceptualizing state intervention as an institutional arrangement; second, by delineating a broad range of social performances at the nation-state level to allow for a better appreciation of the complexities of institutional arrangements; and third, by linking the institutional arrangements of state intervention with social performance to clarify the logics of state and privatized institutional arrangements.

Conceptualizing State Intervention

State intervention in the delivery of medical services is an extremely complex phenomenon, and there are many ways to conceptualize it and to measure its effects. In this analysis, we draw useful insights from the vast literature on complex organizations (Hall, 1977; Chandler, 1966, 1977; Zey-Ferrel, 1979; Mintzberg, 1979; Hage, 1980). The specific perspective we borrow maintains that a critical dimension for describing the institutional arrangement of an organization is the distribution of power along a hierarchy, or its degree of centralization. We also borrow from the perspective of contingency theory in the organizational literature in order to conceptualize how state intervention affects the performance of medical delivery systems. In other words, the performance of medical systems is contingent on how power is distributed in the system (Lawrence and Lorsch, 1967; Perrow, 1967; Mintzberg, 1979; Hage, 1980, chap. 3).

By thinking about state intervention as a form of centralization, we are essentially asking about the degree to which the power to coordinate the activities of a society's medical system is concentrated in the state. Although it is hypothetically possible for the medical system of a country to be highly centralized in the private sector, this type of institutional arrangement has not existed in the history of any Western country (see Figure 1.1). It is important to note, however, that the centralization of the delivery system and the degree of state control over a delivery system are not identical. It is theoretically possible for all of a country's medical system to be in the state sector but to be controlled at the local level—hence to be quite decentralized. Hypothetically, the most centralized medical system is the one in which most critical deci-

Locus of control

Degree of centralization	public	private
low	local government control	market-oriented types of control (for-profit and nonprofit arrangements)
high	centralized state hierarchy	oligopolistic and monopolistic arrangements*

*Whereas privatized monopolistic arrangements may exist at the local level, these arrangements rarely exist in the medical area for a nation as a whole.

Figure 1.1. Dimensions for Understanding State Intervention

sions are located at the national level, and the most decentralized system is the one in which many decision-making points exist in the private sector. Although we have borrowed the term *centralization* from the literature on complex organizations, our interest is specifically with a dimension we label "centralized control under state auspices."

Medical delivery systems are extremely complex, and there are many dimensions through which the state may intervene in its efforts to affect system performance. Some of these dimensions are highly correlated; others are quite independent. Perhaps the most consequential involve sources of revenue, appointment of personnel, and setting the prices of medical services (Hollingsworth and Hanneman, 1984; Meyer and Scott, 1983). We have chosen to differentiate between two basic areas of state intervention: decisions about funding and decisions about the setting of prices and the appointment of personnel. On the basis of considerable study of national medical delivery systems, it is our judgment that these two dimensions capture most of the variation in state intervention among medical delivery systems studied here. For example, a system in which the state provides funding for medical services but makes no effort to control or coordinate prices or the appointment of personnel will perform differently from one in which the state also appoints personnel and controls prices. In the contemporary period, various levels of government in the United States have intervened in funding medical care but have exercised considerably less control over the appointment of personnel and the setting of prices. Most of these decisions have been made in the private sector. The National Health Service in Great Britain, in contrast, displays strong central government control in all three areas. In short, centralization is a multidimensional variable, as our research must reflect.

We must also keep in mind that the degree of state intervention is not static. During the past century, governments in all four countries studied here have generally expanded their functions, increasing their intervention in medical care as in other areas. As part of this trend, the number of functions performed solely at one level of government has declined (Hollingsworth and Hanneman, 1984; Fesler, 1965; Maddick, 1960; Haider, 1971; Farkas, 1971).

This long-term trend toward greater concentration of power in the hands of a centralized state partly results from pressures on the state to help bring about certain outcomes and performances. As various interest groups have campaigned for their preferred utilities, the state has intervened to arbitrate conflicts of values among different groups. Although our research does address the dynamics leading to state intervention, our framework leads to new insights about how the state mediates the effects of other social forces on the performance of medical care delivery systems.

Medical System Performance

The task of conceptualizing the performance of medical systems at the national level is not easy. Fortunately, we can draw on a long tradition in the organizational literature. Sociologists, for example, usually view complex organizations as rationalizing efforts to achieve specific goals, such as the manufacture of goods or the provision of services (Hage and Aiken, 1970). Economists sensitize us to goals that most organizations seek to achieve. For example, organizations, including medical systems, seek to produce outputs (treatments or improvements in health) and to acquire inputs (finance, technology, etc.). Other important dimensions of organizational performance include those which sociologists emphasize, such as the distribution of outputs (especially the degree of equality in the distribution of services); processes of innovation, adaptation, and change of systems; and processes determining the setting of organizational goals and evaluation of performance. We look first at the most familiar of these performance dimensions: levels of health and costs. Then we turn our attention to the somewhat less familiar organizational performances of equality, innovation, and "social" efficiency.

Levels of Health

A basic goal of medical delivery systems is to produce better health. In evaluating the effectiveness of a specific program or a single organization, one might count the number of cures or the number of treatments. To understand national systems and how they change, however, we must consider a much larger social context. Thus, while many factors influence levels of health, societal health is a crucial criterion by which to evaluate the performance of national medical systems.

Cross-national and cross-temporal measures of morbidity and disability and, if possible, even some measure of societal well-being would be invaluable in describing the complex phenomenon of societal health. Unfortunately, however, such data do not uniformly exist from nation to nation throughout the period under study. We therefore rely heavily on mortality data, for it is reasonable to assume that as age-standardized mortality rates decline, citizens have more productive lives and the society is in better health. Even if age-standardized death rates are not ideal measures for levels of health, they are highly useful indicators for cross-temporal and cross-national analysis. For comparisons across nations in the contemporary period or for comparisons within a delivery system, mortality would not be sufficient, but through the broad sweep of time since 1890 in four varied societies, age-sex standardized mortality rates give a sound general measure of societal health and physical well-being (Preston, 1976).

Costs

Most highly industrialized societies during the past two decades have become increasingly concerned with an impending fiscal crisis of the state. In response, concern with containing expenditures has grown in one sector after another. Because medical expenditures have risen more rapidly than those in most sectors, the need to control these costs has gained high priority in most Western countries.

The proportion of societal resources devoted to medical care is a basic aspect of system performance, as well as a key current policy issue. As with levels of health, many factors affect the costs of medical care, and variation in cost performance over time and in different places provides an useful insight into many of the processes by which institutional arrangements affect societal outcomes.

The cost performance of national medical systems is intricately connected with the boundaries of the system. Here, we have not included all activities related to health but have confined our attention to personal medical considerations. Thus, we have excluded collective public health measures, such as public sanitation and water supply and more general efforts to maintain a better social and physical environment, but we have included preventive medical measures administered at the individual level, such as vaccinations. We have included the costs of those activities which are clearly medical in nature, for example, the costs of physicians, nurses, drugs, general and specialized hospitals. Thus, our strategy for estimating medical costs is rather inclusive.

We focus on that part of medical systems which is most immediately concerned with the reduction of mortality. We do not mean to imply that the only important cost-performance issue in medical care is expenditure on this restricted range of services, any more than we would suggest that mortality is the sole issue of concern in assessing system performance. The focus on medical expenditure simply allows us one reasonably comparable and undeniably important basis on which to compare performance.

Other Performances

The first major work on social indicators dealt with outputs and their costs at the nation-state level (Sheldon and Moore, 1968) but did not consider other important kinds of social performance. Increasingly, individuals and groups are concerned about the nature of social institutions and how responsive they are to human needs (Bell, 1973). Because citizens want to know how well their society is performing, a list of performances should reflect the kinds of needs or benefits different segments of the population desire.

Whereas economists measure economic benefits, we wish to measure social benefits. One of many possible ways to develop an appropriate list of "social" performances is to focus on the issues around which conflict arises. Ideally such a list would include (1) things most people, especially the major interest groups of the society, want; (2) objectives that seem to pose dilemmas because they are difficult to achieve simultaneously; and (3) ideas relevant to existing paradigms. This last point is not trivial, for in demonstrating a new analytical paradigm for policy analysis, we want to build upon and synthesize previous scholarly work. By choosing performances that provide the basis for social conflict, we are in fact preserving some aspects of the traditional approach concerned with which interest group won and why and what various interest groups wanted. At the same time, we are expanding on a strategy that parallels present scholarship on program evaluation and cost-benefit analysis, although the costs and benefits on which we focus are social rather than economic.

Innovativeness, social efficiency, and equality are three performances that satisfy our three criteria. Of course, each of these performances is complicated and needs some elaboration. By *innovativeness*, we mean the speed with which a medical delivery system adopts new technologies, services, or programs and diffuses them. By *social efficiency*, we mean how much output is achieved relative to cost—that is, the attainment of a certain level of health at some per capita cost (Hage, Hollingsworth, and Hanneman, 1981). And by *equality*, we mean several things: how much access there is to medical facilities among social classes and income groups, how equitably medical resources are distributed among regions, and how much variation there is in levels of health among social classes and income groups (Hollingsworth, 1981).

Innovativeness

Medical knowledge and technology have advanced rapidly since 1890, but some countries have responded more quickly and completely than others to these advances. Here, we try to specify the circumstances that expedite or impede adoption of technological innovations in specific countries and to explain why innovations diffuse more rapidly in some societies than in others. We will not, however, be concerned with differences among countries in the rate of production of new knowledge or with organizational innovations.

For reasons that we will examine shortly, it appears that national medical systems that permit the rapid diffusion of technical innovations tend to be more costly and less egalitarian. As technology becomes more complex, expensive, and specialized, policies on the adoption of innovations often generate sharply divided opinions. Therefore, an analysis of system innovativeness provides useful insights into the effects of state intervention. In subsequent chapters, we examine how variation in the degree of state intervention influences the diffusion of a variety of innovations, from low-cost, highly efficacious ones demanded by almost everyone to expensive, highly complex ones, which only a few people need. We must also consider how the density and specialization of medical personnel affect the innovativeness of medical delivery systems if we are to understand the impact of state intervention on the adoption and diffusion of new technologies.

Social Efficiency

We use the term *social efficiency* to distinguish a kind of efficiency that is consistent with the sociological literature. For us, social efficiency is broadly concerned with the ratio between the output performance of the entire society and a societal effort. The socially efficient sytstem is one that maximizes levels of health with the least expenditures. Thus, we are interested in the performance of the entire institutional sector of a society, rather than either the cost-benefit or the "technical" efficiency of a particular program or organization. For example, two societies that have similar "levels of health" but spend very different sums of money on medical care would be judged to have substantially different levels of social efficiency.

Economists assume that a medical system is efficient when the most valuable thing it does not do is less valuable than the least valuable thing that it does. They argue that medical resources are efficiently utilized when they cannot be reallocated for alternative strategies of care to attain a more desirable medical outcome. Those assumptions are very difficult to operationalize, however. In our study of social efficiency, by contrast, we rely on a single, somewhat global index (see Chapter 6; Aaron and Schwartz, 1984; 79–89; Williams, 1978).

Interest groups are often sharply divided on the question of how to allocate the social investment in medical care. Some groups place greater emphasis on highly individualized and specialized services; others stress cost containment.

The organizational literature suggests that there is a trade-off between innovativeness and efficiency (Hage, 1965, 1980; Perrow, 1967), and the same insight would seem to apply to the medical systems of entire countries. Providing specialized and individualized services, rather than the same program for everyone, is often more costly for the same level of output. Some innovations may lead to greater social efficiency—for example, low-cost vaccines to prevent various diseases.

Nevertheless, innovations in social services often tend to increase costs while producing only modest improvements in well-being. Indeed, production functions operate very differently in social services from the way they do in manufacturing industries, where new technology is often labor saving.

The institutional arrangements of national medical systems, as well as their social context, may strongly predispose systems toward policy choices that increase costs more than they improve health. In this book we strive to understand some of the processes leading to these choices, especially the role of state intervention and privatization.

According to the human-capital thesis of E. F. Denison (1962, 1967, 1974) and others, increases in skills lead to higher productivity. Social efficiency is not the same as productivity as the economists measure it, but we are concerned with a similar question: whether more physicians and higher levels of specialization produce more or less social efficiency.

Equality

There are several ways of conceptualizing equality, and we discuss four here. The first, equality of rights, is not particularly relevant to the cases we will examine here, but some systems are legally segregated and accord differential treatment to specified social groups. The second, equality of access to a particular good, may not exist even though everyone may have an equal right to the good. The third, regional equality concerns the geographical distribution of the good. Resources may be more concentrated in some regions than others, usually implying, of course, inequality of access by various groups. The last, equality of results, may be most difficult to achieve. In spite of equality in other areas, all social groups may not have equal life chances or the same levels of health.

Analysis of the consequences of state intervention is especially interesting with regard to equality. Many of the most controversial debates in government policy have focused explicitly on this issue. In the United States, for example, the Medicaid and Medicare programs are examples of how the state has tried to provide services to specific categories of people who would otherwise have considerably less access to care. The debates about equality are often very intense not only because they place the interests of different groups into direct conflict but also because achieving greater equality frequently has other costs. A system that maximizes innovativeness, for example, may give lower priority to equal access. A system that gives priority to highly specialized and individualized services is likely to be very costly and to rank low on our measure of social efficiency, as well as equality of access. Thus, a commitment to equality may conflict with other goals of the medical system.

Performance Mixes

There is considerable consensus on how to value the performance of medical systems. In all four countries under study most people desire high levels of health, low costs, innovativeness, social efficiency, and equality. These goals, however, tend to be somewhat incompatible and difficult to achieve simultaneously, and social groups differ sharply about the ranking of these performances. Such conflicts of preference underlie many, if not all, of the specific policy debates about medical care. Systems make choices, and one of our central concerns is to understand the consequences of state intervention, investment in human capital, and the complexity of medical technology for these choices. In the concluding chapter we discuss how alterations in state intervention and human capital might influence the mix of system performance.

The Impact of State Intervention on System Performance

The coordination of medical care by the state has substantial implications for system performance. Max Weber (1947) developed the argument that the concentration of power produces better coordination and more rational administration, leading in turn to increased output and lower unit costs. Weber maintained that the tighter discipline and control characteristic of hierarchical forms of coordination lead to greater predictability, to a greater rationalization of the system. As activities become routinized, they become better coordinated and more efficient. This argument has been further developed by other organization theorists (Hage, 1965, 1980; Perrow, 1967; Price, 1968). It has also been modified and advanced by scholars in business and political economy (Mintzberg, 1979; Chandler, 1966, 1977; Hollingsworth and Lindberg, 1985). Various scholars have argued that centralized systems tend to be concerned more with the quantity of production than with the quality (Burns and Stalker, 1961; Price, 1968; Perrow, 1967; Hage, 1980; Piore and Sabel, 1984; Chandler, 1966, 1977; Hollingsworth and Lindberg, 1985).

Weber's theory is at variance with neoclassical economics, which maintains that coordination by the invisible hand of the marketplace should produce better levels of health and lower unit costs. Some economists, to be sure, have suggested that hierarchical coordination (public or private) may produce lower costs, but only under certain circumstances (Williamson, 1975, 1985; Aoki, 1988). We explore these ideas in greater detail in the chapters that follow; here, we present one observation. The experience of the United States suggests that the logic of a decentralized, privatized system of coordinating of medical care tends to produce substantial duplication of services. The experience of the National Health Service in Britain suggests that centralized state coordination tends to reduce duplication and hold down costs. Apparently, shifting decision making from the private to the public sector and from the local to the central government leads to greater productivity and reduced costs in medical delivery systems. This is quite a strong statement, particularly considering the prevailing arguments in favor of privatizing many social services in the Reagan-Thatcher era. In Chapters 3 and 4 we will return in greater detail to these questions.

In social services, hierarchical structures reveal a preference for social efficiency, standardization, cost containment, and increasing the volume of production, corresponding to the mechanical organizational structure identified by Tom Burns and G. M. Stalker (1961). At the opposite end of the continuum is the decentralized organic structure, whose logic leads to quite different performance preferences. In the organic model, more critical decisions are made at lower levels and there is much more flexible leadership. Delivery systems that display this type of institutional arrangement are likely to emphasize technological innovativeness and quality over quantity, and to place less emphasis on cost containment and efficiency.

Theorists have sought to understand why more decentralized control predisposes a system in these directions. Long ago, Chester Barnard (1946) noted that when power is concentrated in the hands of an elite, new ideas are often vetoed because they threaten the distribution of power and status. Others (Burns and Stalker, 1961; Chandler, 1977) have demonstrated that dispersed power is associated with increased innovativeness because those who are most competent to manage innovative projects will vary from project to project. Jerald Hage (1965, 1980) and J. Rogers Hollingsworth (1986) have suggested that decentralized decision making often leads to joint decision making, which is more innovative. Ideas are developed and altered, modified and augmented when there are competing teams or multiple teams of specialists. A dispersed distribution of power increases the probability that there will be at least one person, organization, research center, or hospital willing to take the risk of an innovation (Ben-David, 1971).

When decision making is concentrated at the highest levels of a system, the tendency to frown upon innovations is joined by the tendency to emphasize the quantity of production and to maximize efficiency. Unit costs are often reduced by increasing volume and standardizing services. But because centralized structures have strong preferences for standardization, once a decision is made to adopt a particular innovation, it is much more rapidly implemented throughout the system than it would be in a decentralized structure.

The organizational literature provides little guidance for understanding the relationship between state intervention and equal distribution of services. Fortunately, other scholars have addressed this subject (for references see Hollingsworth, 1982, 1986). In many cases, the state intervenes in the delivery of medical services in direct response to rising public demand for greater access to care. A high degree of state intervention, motivated by popular pressure for the provision of more services at lower costs, tends to produce a mix of medical services more accessible to all social groups. State hierarchies, by gaining control over medical personnel, sources of funding, and prices of services, are also in a position to dictate where hospitals will be constructed, where professionals may or may not practice, how much the medical system may charge consumers, and how many professionals and specialists there may be. State mechanisms tend to be derived from political considerations, whereas market mechanisms tend to be derived from profit considerations.

Much of the persisting policy debate about the pros and cons of privatization revolves around the propensity for systems centralized under the auspices of the state to differ in their performance from privatized (and less centralized) systems (Friedman, 1955; Levin, 1970; Goldthorpe, 1984: chap. 13). We believe that delivery systems centralized under state auspices are more likely to standardize programs and services, thus considerably cutting unit costs. State systems, however, are also more sensitive to political pressures and may provide more total services to low-income populations, than would be produced by private systems.

Although centralized systems under state auspices tend to promote higher levels of social efficiency, they also might be expected to be less innovative. The exclusion of particular interest groups from the decision-making process, the reliance on public funding, and the avoidance of specialized services make innovation appear costly and unnecessary (Robinson and Kuhlman, 1967; Krueger and Wallisch-Prinz, 1972; Husen, 1969a, 1969b; Paulston, 1968; Meyer and Scott, 1983: chap. 11; Hollingsworth and Hanneman, 1984). The relationship between state intervention and innovativeness is two dimensional, however. If the state simply provides funding without attempting to control costs or prices, the system is likely to adopt more high-cost technologies than the system that vigorously attempts to control prices and reduce the rate of growth in medical spending.

In Figure 1.2 we provide in visual form a summary of the hypotheses we are testing in this study. Note that as the state provides more funding for medical care without controlling prices and personnel, the costs of medical care increase and the social efficiency of the system declines. On the other hand, if the state intervenes to control prices and personnel, the system tends to spend less and to be more socially efficient.

The degrees and forms of state intervention in medical delivery sys-

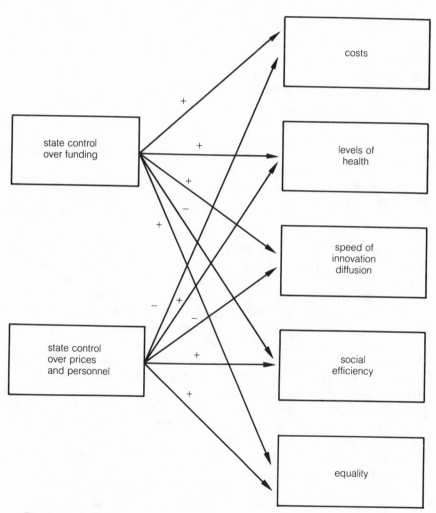

Figure 1.2. Relationship between State Intervention Variables and System Performance

tems are only some of the factors that interact to make some systems more socially efficient than others, some more egalitarian than others, and so on. The changing role of medical knowledge also plays a major role.

A Human-Capital Paradigm in Social Services

State intervention, of course, does not itself produce medical care. The state merely coordinates (or does not coordinate) the combination of human and physical capital by which treatments are applied to patients. To understand why systems perform differently in different places and at different times, we must take account of such "factors of production" as investment in human capital, and how they vary and change.

The organizational literature from which we have borrowed theoretical insights considers the degree of professional training and the complexity of the division of labor just as important in shaping institutional performance as the degree of centralized control over decisions. Both the quantity and quality of the human capital have significant effects on the performance of institutions. These consequences are especially significant in those institutions that provide highly specialized, labor-intensive human services, such as medical care.

During the past eighty years, physicians have moved increasingly from the model of the general practitioner to the model of the specialist (Starr, 1982; Hollingsworth, 1986; Stevens, 1966, 1971). There has also been considerable growth in paramedical specialties and increasing specialization among nurses (Melosh, 1982). The psychiatric nurse has been joined by the x-ray technician, occupational therapist, and so forth. These massive changes in the division of labor in medical delivery systems are highly consequential for system performance.

The causes of this transformation of the division of labor, this movement toward greater and greater specialization, and the ever-expanding number of people in medical delivery systems lie in the growth of knowledge and technology. In the manufacturing sector of the economy, it is often the case that new technology replaces workers. But new technology in the medical sector tends to require new specialists, both professional and subprofessional. Technologies that treat but do not actually cure a given illness tend not to save labor but to generate it. And as popular belief in the capacity of medical technology to cure disease and relieve discomfort has grown dramatically, so has demand for services.

The body of knowledge attached to a delivery system is difficult to conceptualize and, perhaps for that reason, not frequently discussed. The expansion of knowledge is more than merely the accumulation of books in libraries. Much of it exists in skills and know-how that are passed from one generation to the next through apprenticeship or training programs. Some of it consists of practical experience, intuition, art—what is frequently described as clinical judgment.

The complexity of the division of labor in medical care and the quantity and quality of human capital resources are difficult to index adequately. In this book we most frequently use the density of physicians per unit population and the proportion of specialists among them as our indicators. In themselves, these measures can hardly present an exhaustive picture of the dramatic changes in the nature of medical care since 1890. As indicators of the more complex processes, however, they can well reflect differences through time and in several countries.

It is a commonplace of economic theory that specialization increases output and thus reduces unit costs by enhancing productivity, and in some economic sectors, this theory is borne out. In the human services, however, especially the medical sector, specialization does not work in quite the same way. Specialists in human services are frequently added not so much to increase the quantity as to improve the quality of services. There is no necessary gain in the number of clients or patients served, except insofar as improvement in quality leads to greater demand for more services and to higher levels of health. If an increase in specialization does not necessarily lead to an increase in volume in medical delivery systems, it does tend to change the quality of services and to increase cost. Thus specialization may, in some human service activities, actually reduce "technical" (that is, the number of units of output per unit of input) efficiency.

As medical systems become more differentiated and as the number of specialists increases, serious coordination problems occur (Blau, 1970), which may drive up prices. The ratio of administrative to staff personnel tends to rise with increasing specialization, for example, and it becomes necessary to decide how high it should be permitted to rise. Likewise, it must be decided how many places should have specialists, what kind of specialists, how many, and how they should be organized and financed. Specialists, who must have more training, tend to charge more for their services and to make more money (Hage, 1965, 1974; Starr, 1982; Friedman and Kuznets, 1945). Moreover, specialization generates more support staff and increases the need for more physical capital in treatment (Stevens, 1971; Hollingsworth, 1983). For a number of reasons, then, it is reasonable to expect that increased specialization in medical care has substantial consequences for system expenditures.

Increased expenditures, of course, are not the only consequence of increased complexity and human capital investments in medical care.

The quantity and quality of output are also affected. Though there is limited research on the relationship between specialization and quality of care in medical systems over time and among nations, research at the organizational level is suggestive. An interesting example is the Teamsters Union study of hospital care (Trussel, Morehead, and Erlich, 1961), which found that increasing the proportion of specialists in hospitals improved the quality of care. Also suggestive are studies showing that the more open-heart, vascular, or other surgical procedures a team performs, the lower the mortality rate among their patients (Fuchs, 1986; Luft, Bunker, and Enthoven, 1979). The increasing complexity and professional density of medical care, then, might be expected to have major consequences for the quality, if not the quantity of treatment delivered.

There has been considerable work at the organizational level on the relationship between specialization and innovation (Hage and Aiken, 1970; Aiken and Hage, 1971; Zaltman, Duncan, and Holbek, 1973; Hage and Dewar, 1973; Moch, 1976). This literature suggests a strong causal linkage between professional density and the speeed with which new techniques are adopted and diffused through an entire society. Professionalization and specialization influence the adoption of innovations by several routes. In general, higher levels of professional training lead to greater knowledge about new discoveries and an interest in seeking them out. The literature on the diffusion of innovation (Rogers, 1962; Zaltman, Duncan, and Holbek, 1973; Meyer and Scott, 1983, chap. 11) demonstrates that the gatekeepers for innovation are individuals who read more, actively monitor their environment, and thus seek out new inventions. Organizations that have high professional density are more likely to develop new ideas, more likely to hear about innovations elsewhere, and more likely to adopt them. We expect that these same tendencies characterize the behavior of medical organizations, as well as the behavior of a nation's entire medical system.

Whereas the density of professionalization and the level of specialization enhance quality and innovativeness, they may on balance decrease social efficiency. Again, it is important to emphasize that the medical sector does not behave the same way as the manufacturing sector. Technological innovations in manufacturing are usually adopted to increase technical efficiency. In the medical area, technological innovations (embodied in both human and physical capital) generally do not increase the quantity of treatment (output) per unit cost, though the quality may be markedly improved. Many medical innovations are socially efficient because they greatly improve population health despite increased costs. A technology that is quite efficacious in preventing or curing a disease may markedly increase social efficiency. But in medicine, there are many "half-way technologies," as Lewis Thomas calls them, which are only diagnostic, palliative, or aimed at maintaining patients who suffer a noncurable disease. They neither cure nor prevent disease and are usually quite expensive (Thomas, 1977). Considerable expenditure on such technologies may not be socially efficient.

Advances in medical technology which improve society's level of health may simultaneously drive up the costs of medical care. Medical practitioners—particularly specialists—place strong value on innovations and new technologies. National medical systems dominated by professional specialists are likely to support changes that expand costs more rapidly than they improve general population health, resulting in lower social efficiency than systems dominated by governments.

Neither the literature on organizations nor the literature on the nation-state has much to say about the relationship between equal distribution of services and increases in the levels of professionalization and specialization. On balance, however, we believe that increases in the level of specialization reduce equality in access to care and in the spatial distribution of resources.

As specialization increases in market-oriented economies specialists tend to concentrate in proximity to upper-income populations. As a consequence, the higher the level of specialization, the greater the access of upper-income groups to complex medical technology. This factor accounts for much of the difference in the kind of medical care given upper- and lower-income groups. For example, in the United States, even though the federal government has financed medical care for the elderly, those with higher incomes have tended to receive care more often from specialists and in elite hospitals, and lower income groups have tended to receive care more often from general practitioners in crowded public hospitals (Hollingsworth, 1986; Hollingsworth and Hollingsworth, 1987; Davis, 1975).

The impact of specialization in narrowing the disparity in levels of health among social groups may be even less salutary. Specialization not only may lead to differential access to quality care but may encourage the development of technology for the treatment of upper-income groups. Given the substantial inequalities in life styles (for example, income, wealth, nutrition, housing, etc.) in the general population, unless medical care is biased in a compensatory direction, there are likely to be substantial variations in levels of health across social classes and income groups (Hollingsworth, 1981, 1986).

Figure 1.3 summarizes our hypotheses about the relationship between the two human capital variables and the performance of national medical systems, and in subsequent chapters we attempt to assess their validity.

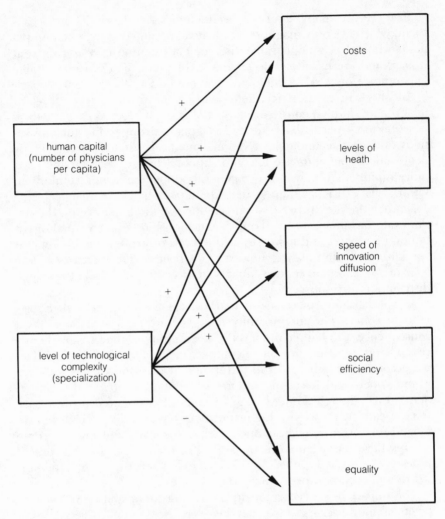

Figure 1.3. Effects of Human Capital and Technological Complexity on System Performance

The Societal Context and System Performance

Our main concerns in the remainder of this book are with the effects of
state intervention, investment in human capital, and the complexity of
medical technology on system performance. In focusing on these
"structures" (that is, forms and degrees of state intervention, investment in human capital, and complexity of medical technology) and
their consequences for "performance" (that is, equality, cost, level of

health, social efficiency, etc.), we are following in a long tradition of macrosociological research. The cross-temporal and cross-national differences in the performances of the medical systems of Britain, France, Sweden, and the United States between 1890 and 1970 are, in large part, the consequence of these "structural" factors. It is also important to recognize, however, that medical systems and the state do not operate in isolation. The performance of medical systems and the structures that influence these performances are constrained and shaped by larger historical and societal factors, which we will explore in the chapters that follow. For the moment it will suffice to identify some of the most important of these other factors.

Scholars have often found that the size of a system and the spatial distribution and density of its actors may influence the division of labor, the method of coordination, and consequently the performance (Hanneman and Hollingsworth, 1984; Hollingsworth and Hanneman, 1984; Hollingsworth, 1982, 1986; Meyer, 1972; Dahl and Tufte, 1973; Hage, 1980). Social service delivery systems in large democratic societies have been somewhat more decentralized than those in smaller democratic societies (Hollingsworth and Hanneman, 1984). Hence, all other things being equal, one would expect a country the size of the United States to have a medical delivery system somewhat more decentralized—and hence more privatized—than that in Great Britain or Sweden.

The relationship between system size and decentralization of social systems is not as simple as it might seem, however. If we compare the systems of nations at any one time, societies with larger delivery systems (like the United States) do have less centralized administration, but within a large society over time, the picture is somewhat different. In the United States, for example, the size of the delivery system has increased markedly since World War II, and administrative centralization has also increased. This is not to say that system size has no effect on administrative centralization. Indeed, we believe that it does. Nevertheless, the operation of other factors (increasing medical complexity, state intervention, etc.) may over time outweigh the effects of system size.

Size of country is also linked to social heterogeneity: the greater the size of the country, the more diverse and heterogeneous the society and the greater the lines of cleavage among consumer groups. Thus, the larger the country, the more difficult it is for lower income groups to mobilize sufficient power to influence the medical delivery system (Stephens, 1979; Hollingsworth and Hanneman, 1982; Hollingsworth, 1986). That is to say, the more fragmented the power of consumer groups, the less potential there is to focus state power to provide more open access to a medical delivery system. Size of country is an important variable influencing the structure and role of the state, which in turn influences the performance of the medical delivery system. Because there is less access to medical delivery systems in larger and less-centralized countries, we can expect such countries to have lower levels of health—all other things being equal. Because size of country influences the level of centralization under state auspices, we would expect that it also has indirect effects on innovativeness, costs, and social efficiency.

A substantial body of literature links increases in levels of income and wealth, as well as various indicators of modernization (for example, levels of literacy, communication, and the proportion of the population age sixty-five and over) to rising demand for more medical professionals and specialization, which leads to higher levels of state involvement. As medical technology becomes more efficacious—or as the society believes that medical technology becomes more efficacious—and as the costs of medical technology mount, the public pressures the state to increase its responsibility in providing medical services.

Since income, wealth, and modernization are so positively associated and intricately linked with one another, we will, in the chapters that follow, combine them into a single measure which we call the index of social development. Increases in social development have led to the development of new knowledge, which in turn has generated demand for more professionalization and specialization.

Though the institutional characteristics of medical delivery systems mediate the effects of social development on performance, the level of social development does have some independent effect. Thus, a major task in our research is to distinguish the effects of such institutional variables as centralization under state auspices, level of investment in human capital, and technological complexity from the effects of social development on the performance of the medical delivery system. Otherwise, we would not know whether our institutional variables are spurious, and changes in performance are actually caused by social development. We have therefore designed our research to determine the independent effect of each of our variables on performance.

For example, most of the variables in our social development index accelerate the diffusion of innovations throughout an entire delivery system (Hollingsworth, Hage, and Hanneman, 1978). Previous work has suggested that social development has an independent effect on the speed of diffusion but is also mediated by the medical delivery system. Irrespective of the level of social development, a highly centralized delivery system that wishes to prevent the adoption and diffusion of an innovation may succeed in doing so (ibid.; Hollingsworth, 1986).

Most of the variables in our social development index lead to higher levels of spending on medical care. Many studies demonstrate that the higher the gross national product of a society, the more resources it can afford to spend on medical care, and therefore the more it actually spends. Moreover, increases in levels of education, communication, and the proportion of the population age sixty-five and over generate more demand for medical care, leading to higher levels of medical expenditures. Thus, for all these reasons, we expect the social development index to lead to higher expenditures on medical care. Again, an interesting problem in our research will be to assess the independent effects of social development on spending and to determine how the institutional structure of the medical delivery system limits medical spending.

Although few scholars have worked with the concept of social efficiency at the level of the nation-state, in a previous publication (Hage, Hollingsworth, and Hanneman, 1981) we reported our finding that increases in the level of social development lead to decreases in social efficiency, though the level of centralization may constrain the decrease. Thomas McKeown and others (McKeown, 1976a and b; McKeown, Record, and Turner, 1975; Powles, 1973) have tended to downplay the importance of medical delivery systems in bringing about lower mortality rates, attributing them instead to a higher standard of living. Because the policy implications are so important, we address this issue in subsequent chapters. Specifically, we agree that increases in the standard of living have caused a decline in twentieth-century mortality rates, but we maintain that most of the effect of the improvements in the standard of living on mortality has been mediated by the medical delivery system. This finding, of course, is not a rejection but an important refinement and extension of McKeown's position.

Societal development affects the performance of the medical delivery system in still another way: by influencing the level and form of state intervention. Because social development leads to greater political awareness and political mobilization among consumer groups, which demand state intervention to equalize access to medical care or to further other goals (Almond and Powell, 1966; Hollingsworth, 1971; Grew, 1978), social development has a modest propensity to generate more egalitarian medical delivery systems.

We examine how social development affects system characteristics in Chapter 2, providing qualitative and quantitative data. Our analysis in Chapters 3 through 7 stresses the interplay of social development, state intervention, and human capital, seeking to understand how the structural characteristics of the medical delivery system mediate the influences of social development. We use both path analysis and qualitative data to examine the direct and indirect effects of these variables on performance.

As we attempt to discover the consequences of privatization or state intervention for national medical systems, we hope to contribute to the various new forms of institutional analysis now prevalent in sociology, economics, political science, as well as in historical scholarship. Some proponents of medical reform believe that privatization is more likely to be socially efficient, but this may well be a myth that has gained credibility because few study the impact of state intervention on social efficiency, especially at the nation-state level. Because most scholarship about efficiency has tended to focus on a specific program in a particular organization, we know very little about the social efficiency of national systems. And most scholars who have studied the state and social services have been more concerned with analyzing why the state intervenes than with understanding the consequences of state action.

Furthermore, little has been done to assess a broader range of consequences. The efficacy of one institutional arrangement or another—private or market-oriented system versus state hierarchy—should be evaluated not only in terms of efficiency but in terms of effectiveness (defined by the level of health or rate of mortality), equality of access, and innovativeness. One of our objectives is to debunk efficiency as the sole criterion for judging a social system, although admittedly the current concerns about medical costs have made cost control a critical issue.

Another objective is to begin developing a theory about the logic of privatization and the logic of state intervention, at least in the social services. How resources are allocated and coordinated tells us a great deal about why services perform well in some sectors of the economy and not others. Chapters 3 through 8 treat this issue as a recurring theme.

In this chapter, we have attempted to present a new paradigm of comparative macropolicy analysis and to apply it to the performance of national medical systems. We have suggested that when national delivery systems are viewed as analogues to complex organizations, it becomes clear that their degree of "centralization" is a key dimension of variability. In subsequent chapters, we focus on centralization under the auspices of the state, one of the most important changes in how the delivery of medical care has been organized in Western nations. We address the critical question of how variation in the degree of such centralization influences variation in the performance of national medical systems. Because state intervention is by no means the only important force shaping performance over time, we also explore the effect of such variables as investment in human capital and the complexity of medical technology on system performance and how these factors have interacted with state intervention. Finally, neither the changing role of the state nor the impact of technology and specialization can be understood independently of the larger societal forces in which the systems are embedded. We seek to understand how various societal dynamics have interacted with the structure of medical systems and the state to produce changes in system performance.

Insofar as this book can provide some initial answers to these questions, it can open a new agenda for policy research. Our approach should begin to show how state intervention interacts with changing medical knowledge and societal forces to produce changes in medical performance. Only such an analysis can permit a reasonable prediction of the consequences of state or privatized control.

The main body of this book (Chapters 3–7) presents studies of the several system performances we have discussed. In these chapters we engage in a theoretical analysis that connects the societal context, investment in human capital, and state intervention to system performance, and we also provide evidence with which to evaluate our theoretical arguments. The evidence is primarily qualitative and historical, but we also apply statistical analyses as an useful means of formalizing and illustrating the complex causal connections among the forces that have shaped the performance of medical delivery systems.

Because the statistical analyses are intended as illustrative and exploratory, the quantitative arguments should not stand or fall on the evidence they present. The statistical results in subsequent chapters, though suggestive, must be interpreted with some care. In appendixes we discuss the sources of the data, their tranformation, and the strengths and weaknesses of the statistical models and estimation methods underlying the results. The qualitative and statistical analyses are designed to complement each other, providing counterchecks that can be tested.

In the core chapters we are more interested in explicating and evaluating our theory than in providing historical and descriptive accounts of each national medical system. The institutional and historical differences among the systems, which are of great interest and importance, have been explicated by a large body of excellent scholarship, on which we have drawn. Chapter 2 gives those readers unfamiliar with the four cases we examine—Great Britain, France, Sweden, and the United States—an introduction to the evolution of their social contexts, medical systems, and patterns of state intervention between 1890 and 1970. Though the discussion is confined to those trends and variables which will be discussed in the remainder of the book, those readers interested primarily in the theoretical issues of how state intervention and privatization, investment in human capital, and levels of social development influence system performance may wish to by-pass Chapter 2 and turn directly to Chapters 3 through 8.

2

FOUR NATIONAL
MEDICAL SYSTEMS

Since 1890 the institutional arrangements of the medical systems in Europe and North America have undergone transformation. In the chapters that follow, we attempt to identify some of these changes as we test the general propositions put forth in the previous chapter. First, however, we want to describe in broad outline the medical systems of France, Great Britain, Sweden, and the United States as they have evolved in response to societal changes from 1890 to 1970, to see what similarities and dissimilarities we can discover in these four institutional histories. Space considerations, as well as the theses of this book, will keep our account focused on the growth of state intervention, increased investment in human capital, and social development. Through these three categories we examine the independent variables to be used in the analysis to come, describing how they differ in four countries and how they have changed in eight decades. In the course of this discussion, we hope to convey a sense of both the usefulness of these variables and their limitations.

Institutional Patterns of State Coordination and Control

The differences among the four delivery systems in how decisions are made and activities coordinated are far too complex and subtle to be delineated by the common categorization of medical systems as either "socialized" or "free-market." By 1970 all four systems were coordinated by the state to some extent, though the specific components of coordination varied. Administrative controls existed at different levels (national, regional, local) in the several systems. Some of the administrative mechanisms were public (for example, the British National Health Service), one was quasi-public (the French Social Insurance systems), and one was quite private (the United States tended to use many more market-oriented mechanisms of coordination).

It is not possible here to describe in detail the wide variety of coordinative mechanisms and their evolution. By examining a few indicators, however, we can highlight the key differences and similarities among the systems. We have chosen to discuss patterns of ownership, control, and financing of medical care because, although variations in these aspects do not tell the entire story, they do broadly indicate how state coordination has developed in the four systems.

Certainly, the state has become increasingly involved in the coordination of medical care over the past century in most countries of the world. When, how, and to what extent the state has intervened have varied greatly from one country to another, however. In the four countries under study, the state has become more or less important in rationing and equalizing access to care, in controlling the supply and distribution of personnel and physical capital, and in influencing the type of medical services available. In all four countries, financial controls have been among the most important, as state financing of medical care has substantially increased since 1890.

State financial coordination and control can take many forms. The state may manipulate the supply of hospital beds and medical personnel or may determine priorities and prices. For example, state expenditures and subsidies might be used to increase the number of physicians and hospitals and hence to influence the quantity, quality, and price of services available. The state may also intervene more directly by setting prices, by establishing eligibility criteria for care under public programs, and by providing reimbursement schedules. In this book we employ three measures of state financial intervention: control over revenues, prices, and personnel.

Revenues

Table 2.1 indexes in gross form the extent of centralized state funding of medical services in the four nations over time. The index contrasts the proportion of revenues contributed by private sources to that from state sources, including central, regional, and local government

Table 2.1. Index of State Control over Medical Revenues, 1890–1970

Year	United States	Great Britain	France	Sweden
1890	.009	.030	.071	.210
1900	.085	.060	.108	.230
1910	.064	.112	.169	.250
1920	.104	.169	.335	.277
1930	.091	.163	.335	.291
1940	.128	.200	.447	.358
1950	.185	.818	.541	.519
1960	.176	.782	.528	.579
1970	.314	.857	.636	.571

Sources: See Appendix 1.

Note: For methods of constructing this index, see Appendix 2.

authorities, weighted by degree of centralization (See Appendix 2). The general increase evident in this table has been not a uniform progression but a series of discrete steps. In each nation there has been a marked tendency toward increased governmental financing of medical care. Moreover, the timing and extent of governmental financing, as well as the sector of government involved, have varied from nation to nation.

In the United States, local and state governments have provided from 5 to 20 percent of total medical funding since 1900, while federal government expenditures have risen stepwise from less than 1 percent prior to World War I to about 5 percent in the interwar period, to 10 percent in the post–World War II period, to 25 percent during Lyndon Johnson's "Great Society." Today, all forms of state spending represent almost 50 percent of total medical funding.

At the turn of the century, the pattern in Great Britain resembled that in the United States, but it jumped to almost complete governmental financing when the National Health Service began in 1948. The local and regional governmental role has remained relatively constant in Great Britain, providing less than 5 percent of all medical revenues. The involvement of the central government, however, rose from almost zero in the early years of the century to 20 percent during the National Health Insurance period (1912–1948), to approximately 80 percent under the National Health Service.

In 1890 the governments of France and Sweden were already involved in financing medical services. In France revenues from both central and local governments rose together until World War II. Since then, the financial burden has shifted markedly toward the central government. In Sweden already-substantial government spending early in the century was primarily at the subnational level, but during the interwar years, central government financing grew rapidly, so that by 1940 the central and subnational levels of government were each providing about 25 percent of total medical revenues. In the postwar period, funding in Sweden, unlike France, shifted back to subnational levels of government, which by 1970 provided approximately 65 percent of all medical revenues, while the central government provided an additional 25 percent.

Prices and Personnel

In most cases, increases in state financing of medical care have been driven by political demands for more and better care and equal access to it. In the European countries, the expanded role in financing has brought with it considerable state control over medical prices and personnel (see Table 2.2). That is, the state has come to set or limit prices

Table 2.2. Indexes of State Control over Prices and Personnel, 1890–1970

Year	Index	United States	Great Britain	France	Sweden
1890	prices	.008	.030	.234	.633
	personnel	.025	.095	.290	.638
	combined	.000	.090	.363	.908
1900	prices	.085	.060	.245	.635
	personnel	.039	.097	.198	.600
	combined	.061	.092	.295	.877
1910	prices	.064	.112	.333	.637
	personnel	.046	.100	.158	.646
	combined	.053	.129	.319	.917
1920	prices	.104	.321	.501	.639
	personnel	.046	.116	.144	.596
	combined	.079	.276	.414	.877
1930	prices	.053	.338	.565	.648
	personnel	.052	.108	.165	.572
	combined	.050	.280	.473	.862
1940	prices	.104	.370	.626	.698
	personnel	.061	.131	.159	.563
	combined	.090	.320	.508	.888
1950	prices	.105	.830	.676	.728
	personnel	.073	.526	.164	.531
	combined	.101	.941	.543	.880
1960	prices	.100	.823	.683	.719
	personnel	.080	.540	.160	.572
	combined	.103	.948	.545	.908
1970	prices	.092	.882	.763	.649
	personnel	.127	.566	.261	.459
	combined	.138	1.000	.680	.770

Sources: See Appendix 1.

Note: For methods of constructing these indexes, see Appendix 2.

of medical services and has become an employer of medical personnel (the personnel index in Table 2.2 is limited to doctors).

The indexes in Table 2.2 measure direct controls, rather than indirect incentives and market manipulations. Clearly, the three European cases diverge sharply from the United States. In France, Great Britain, and Sweden state control over pricing rose with state contributions to funding, reaching quite high levels by 1970. In the United States, by contrast, not only was the government consistently less involved in financing, but it was even less inclined to fix the prices of medical services.

The pattern of physician employment is somewhat different. In the United States few physicians are government employees, and most of these are employed at the state and local levels. In Great Britain, although an extremely high proportion of doctors are employed by the state under the National Health Service (continuing a long trend of substantial government employment), government control is less centralized than it is in pricing. A sizable proportion of physician employment occurred at the local government level. Moreover, many hospital-based doctors employed by regional hospital authorities had part-time appointments and devoted some time to private practice.

Centralized state control over the employment of physicians in France and Sweden tended to decrease over time—the opposite trend to the United States and Great Britain. Both France and Sweden, as we will see later, were late-developing nations in which the state was a major provider of medical services throughout the nineteenth century. Even so, direct governmental employment of physicians in France never had strong support as public policy, and until the 1960s, most additions to the supply of physicians tended to occur in the private sector. At present, approximately two-thirds of all French physicians are in private practice (American Medical Association, 1976:97–98). The direct public employment of physicians was somewhat more common in Sweden. Between 65 and 75 percent of all Swedish physicians were public employees between 1890 and the 1960s. Centralized state control of Swedish physicians declined between 1910 and 1970 because Sweden increasingly tended to integrate medical care at the subnational or county level (Heidenheimer and Elvander, 1980).

Our empirical investigations have revealed that centralized price control and personnel employment have similar effects on the performance of medical delivery systems. We have therefore combined these two measures into a single index, which we use as one of the two main indicators of state intervention (see Appendix 2).

Table 2.3 presents data on hospital ownership, a particularly important indicator. Through hospital ownership the state can exercise le-

Table 2.3. Percentage of All Beds in Government Hospitals, 1890–1970

Year	United States	England and Wales	France	Sweden
1890	NA	74	91	92
1900	NA	76	88	92
1910	47	77	89	92
1920	47	75	89	92
1930	65	70	86	93
1940	71	64	83	95
1950	71	99	81	94
1960	68	99	74	95
1970	58	99	73	97

Sources: See Appendix 1.

Note: Both chronic- and acute-care facilities are included in these data. In countries where both public and private sectors were sizable, most long-term-care facilities (mental hospitals, tuberculosis hospitals, hospices, etc.) were in the public sector, and most acute-care hospitals were in the private sector.

verage over many aspects of a nation's medical system, for capital-intensive and complex medical technology has tended to be concentrated in hospitals.

The data in Table 2.3 reveal several distinct patterns of response to the demand for hospital care. The Swedish and French cases demonstrate the early involvement of the state in the provision of hospital care, but neither state had a high commitment to providing widespread medical care outside the hospital in the first decades of this century. Since 1890 the systems of France and Sweden have diverged somewhat. In Sweden, government ownership of hospital facilities has persisted with economic development (Heidenheimer and Elvander, 1980), and virtually all hospitals have historically been owned by the state. Moreover, Swedish hospitals have long cared for both inpatients and outpatients, and hospitals have thus played a more prominent role than they have in the other three countries. The long history of hospital ownership has given the Swedish state a strong tradition of involvement in the delivery of medical care (Berg, 1980; Ito, 1980).

In France, where nearly as high a percentage of hospitals were state owned in 1890, the opposite has occurred; the role of the private sector has increased. Beginning in 1901 the French government allowed more and more private hospitals and clinics to be created, especially in areas with few public hospitals. Since the 1940s, the number of privately owned clinics has increased. Nevertheless, a large proportion of French hospitals are still state owned, and the private sector is heavily regulated. In 1980 two-thirds of all beds were in public hospitals, but private hospitals accommodated 50 percent of all patients. In general, private hospitals have tended to be located more in Paris and in the south; public hospitals have been more numerous in the east than in the west. As in most countries, public hospitals have been quite large, averaging six hundred beds, compared to the sixty-bed average for private hospitals.

The story is more complex in Britain. There, hospitals developed as a form of private philanthropy in conjunction with government involvement through the operation of the Poor Law. This mixed pattern persisted into the interwar years, when both the local government and the private sector found it increasingly difficult to finance and upgrade aging hospitals (Abel-Smith, 1964; Hollingsworth and Hollingsworth, 1984; Hollingsworth, 1986). The attempt to centralize the administration of health care by reorganizing the British medical system under the National Health Service in 1948 was partly a response to a crisis in the provision of hospital care. Even under the National Health Service, however, centralized state administrative control over the hospital sector was not complete, for regional and teaching hospital authorities retained some autonomy, and there was limited provision for private, paying patients in publicly owned hospitals.

In this as in other respects, the pattern in the United States has historically diverged from the European examples. In general, more American hospitals have been private; central government ownership has been confined to military hospitals and hospitals on Indian reservations. Most hospitals owned by state governments have been chronic-care institutions (particularly psychiatric facilities). Acute-care hospitals have primarily been of three types: municipally owned, nonprofit, and for-profit institutions (Hollingsworth and Hollingsworth, 1987; Rosenberg, 1987; Stevens, 1989). Whereas the state has been very much involved in coordinating hospital care in Europe, the Americans have chosen a more varied set of strategies.

Taken together, the data on governmental control of medical care through hospital ownership, personnel employment, and financial control reveal four unique management systems. In all countries the state's role has grown since 1890, but because of differences in the nature and extent of state intervention and in the rates of increase, the systems were still substantially different in 1970.

The American system has relied most consistently and most heavily on private-sector mechanisms for coordination. Central, state and local governments have had relatively less involvement in the direct provision of services than in the European cases and have largely restricted their activities to special populations (veterans, minorities, the mentally ill, the handicapped, the elderly, and the poor). Nevertheless, the American governments, especially the federal government, have greatly increased spending on medical care. Yet in general medical expenditures by various levels of government have not been accompanied by extensive state controls over other aspects of medical systems in the United States. In other words, increases in state funding of medical care have not led to an increase in the proportion of physicians employed by government at any level or to rigorous controls over the prices of medical services, though during the 1980s the central government did begin to exercise rigorous price controls for the treatment of hospitalized Medicare patients.

France, like the United States, has shown a propensity to rely on quasi-market forms of coordination, rather than direct governmental administrative control. The French, however, began the twentieth century with much more state ownership of hospitals. The major French efforts toward state coordination of the delivery of medical services have been through financial means, as in the United States, but in France dramatic increases in state funding have brought extensive regulation of prices (National Center for Health Statistics, 1983).

Great Britain in 1890 had an essentially private medical system, but by 1970 state involvement was more pervasive than in any of the other three systems. This transformation occurred in stages as central government policy built on preexisting trends in the sectors of private enterprise and local government, ratifying and rationalizing those trends. State employment of physicians under the National Health Service, for example, was in many ways an extension of the "panel doctor" principle of the earlier National Health Insurance program, which in turn grew out of the even earlier capitation employment of physicians by unions and mutual aid societies. The National Health Service was distinctive in its widespread use of governmental ownership of hospitals and employment of physicians to coordinate medical activity (Honigsbaum, 1979; Hollingsworth, 1986; Stevens, 1966).

In its use of multiple, reenforcing control strategies, the Swedish medical system by 1970 somewhat resembled that of the British National Health Service. Sweden, however, had arrived at its strategy by a quite different historical process, for in 1890 virtually all hospitals and a large proportion of medical personnel were already under governmental control (Heidenheimer and Elvander, 1980).

Investment in Human and Physical Capital

The substantial growth of the four medical systems during the past century reflects a major reallocation of human and physical resources.

Perhaps the most general indicator of this growth is the amount of money spent on medical care in the four countries, data we present in Table 2.4. These figures, in 1938 constant U.S. dollars, represent both operating expenses and capital investment, comprising physician visits as well as purchase of physical stock—whether for hospitals or half-way houses—ranging from computerized axial tomography scanners to thermometers, plant and equipment, and so on. While it is somewhat difficult to get precise cross-temporal and cross-national measurements of spending on medical care, the data in Table 2.4 are careful estimates of the variations in medical expenditures among these four countries. Clearly, all four have proceeded on the path of medicalization, though not at the same pace or in the same pattern.

In the United States, where medical expenditures were higher than in the other nations over the entire period, growth was essentially steady from 1890 to 1960, albeit increasing at a slightly more rapid rate between 1920 and 1950 than earlier. From 1960 to 1970, however, spending nearly doubled, largely because of government intervention, as we will discuss in Chapter 3.

The Swedish pattern was much the same, although spending remained at a much lower level throughout the entire period. The major surge in Swedish allocation of resources to medical care occurred in the 1950s, when the state took on a new role in the funding of medical care. In Great Britain spending was constant during the first decade of the century and declined during the second, before beginning to rise. Exceptionally rapid growth during the thirties slowed during World War II and after, but by the 1960s there was an acceleration in spending. French spending shrank steadily for thirty years to a low point in 1920, then began to grow again, doubling every ten years until growth

Table 2.4. Medical Expenditures per Capita (1938 Constant U.S. Dollars), 1890–1970

Year	United States	Great Britain	France	Sweden
1890	8.41	8.35	5.61	1.51
1900	10.76	8.37	4.99	2.71
1910	14.31	8.39	4.43	3.93
1920	15.55	6.71	3.08	5.59
1930	25.21	9.63	3.63	7.58
1940	29.55	20.37	6.63	14.94
1950	43.37	28.24	14.14	17.44
1960	61.21	36.23	28.85	31.31
1970	119.45	56.87	51.92	69.72

Sources: See Appendix 1.

slowed somewhat in the 1960s (Heidenheimer and Elvander, 1980; Klein, 1983; National Center for Health Statistics, 1983).

Let us use the French case to illustrate how the political and economic environment of a country shapes its medical expenditures. In France the aftermath of World War I was a period of social, political, and economic stagnation, which lasted through the 1920s and 1930s. This stagnation, which also affected education and other systems, severely limited the growth of the French medical system despite the introduction of social security and the absorption of substantial private health insurance funds by the state (Hage, Hanneman, and Gargan, 1989). In large measure the slowdown in medical expenditures was attributable to a lack of investment in new technologies, especially in hospitals (in contrast, the hospital sector in the United States was growing rapidly during the 1920s). In addition, economies of scale permitted the same physical plant to process more patients, keeping per-patient spending low. Indeed, less was spent per patient in 1941 than had been spent in 1901 (Rochaix, 1959). Another factor that kept spending low was the lack of "free" medical care for the dependents of workers, many of whom had some form of third-party coverage after 1930.

After World War II the demand for access to medical care increased dramatically, and two crucial decisions sent spending up. In 1945, the French government centralized the system of paying the medical bills for millions of citizens (Steudler, 1973), and then in 1946 the coalition government removed a major financial barrier by making dependents of workers eligible for publicly funded medical care. An explosion in hospital utilization and medical expenditures ensued. The number of patients in public hospitals had grown slowly from 614,000 in 1888 to 823,000 in 1921. In the next decade the number of patients grew by 50 percent, largely because of the creation of social security in 1928–1930 and also because of the rapid growth in *sociétés des aides mutuelles*, the private insurance societies that were the precursor to the French social security system. Then, from 1944 to 1948, thanks to the eligibility of dependents for public care, the number of patients shot up 54 percent, from 1,082,000 to 1,665,067 patients. In the next five years the number of patients continued to grow, but at a slower pace, to 1,962,875 in 1953 (Rochaix, 1959:224). By 1950, the French nation was funding medical care for most French citizens. The rapid economic growth of the period after World War II made it possible to invest in complex and expensive new technology and to spend more than ever before on medical care.

After 1950 the introduction of the scientific model of medical care continued to drive up costs. For example, the number of laboratory tests grew at the rate of 18 percent per year in the 1960s, x-rays at 13 percent, medical interventions at 13 percent, and surgical procedures at 11 percent. Because of this new reliance on tests and interventions, medical costs more than doubled in the 1950s and nearly doubled in the 1960s. In this way, paradoxically, public spending on medical care helped to make care more expensive for that part of the population who did not qualify for public assistance (Rochaix, 1959; Steudler, 1973; Hatzfeld, 1971; Thorsen, 1974).

France, Great Britain, Sweden, and the United States also differ in the number and distribution of medical practitioners. Table 2.5 presents two aspects of this variant: numbers of physicians and surgeons per 100,000 population and the percentage of specialists among these practitioners. Regarding the first aspect, the picture in the United States from 1890 to 1920 is somewhat clouded. Census reports of the number of physicians actually practicing per unit of population far exceed physician density in the other sample countries and, indeed, probably in every other country of Western Europe or North America. Many of these doctors were relatively untrained apprentices or trained in substandard medical schools (Stevens, 1971). In the European nations, however, the figures more accurately represent fully qualified and fairly well trained doctors. To derive comparable figures for the United States, therefore, we have estimated the number of fully qualified doctors from lists of graduates of reputable medical schools over lengthy periods prior to the date shown.

Despite the two sets of data for the United States, the four nations clearly differ in per capita investment in human capital. If we consider only physicians trained in formal medical schools, the growth pattern in the United States and Great Britain were basically linear, but the two late-developing nations had patterns of very sharp increases in later years. Moreover, the supply of doctors expanded slowly in the first two countries. In the United States from 1920 to 1970, for example, the total number of physicians per capita grew quite modestly, and in Great Britain, physician supply increased by 53 percent; by contrast, physician supply in France and Sweden grew by 155 and 385 percent, respectively, over the same period. In part the difference in the timing in the growth of physician supply is attributable to the later economic development of France and Sweden and to their attempts to "catch up" with the United States and Great Britain. Consistent with this view, the most dramatic increase in France and Sweden actually occurred between 1960 and 1980 (American Medical Association, 1976; Berg, 1984).

While their numbers were increasing, physicians in all four nations were becoming far more sophisticated and differentiated. Doctors became better qualified, and their training more standardized. Before

Table 2.5. Indicators of Human Capital and Medical Complexity, 1890–1970

Year	United States	Great Britain	France	Sweden
	Physicians and surgeons per 100,000 population			
1890	166 (17)*	68	32	17
1900	175 (16)	69	41	22
1910	164 (69)	65	51	23
1920	136 (90)	66	52	28
1930	125	77	61	37
1940	125	88	66	48
1950	145	72	89	69
1960	144	92	105	95
1970	163	101	133	136
1980	201	126	194	220
	Percentage of specialists among physicians			
1890	0.5	2.5	3.2	6.2
1900	1.1	3.1	3.8	10.0
1910	3.6	5.2	3.6	16.0
1920	9.6	7.0	4.8	18.8
1930	17.0	7.8	19.0	33.5
1940	23.5	8.2	24.6	50.1
1950	36.8	24.2	28.7	50.1
1960	57.3	27.2	35.8	55.9
1970	77.0	34.1	42.4	55.7

Sources: See Appendix 1.

*Figures represent the number of physicians in actual practice. In parentheses are numbers of medical school graduates.

1900, there had been a variety of competing modes of treatment, but by the early twentieth century, a single medical model became increasingly dominant in each country (Starr, 1982; Rothstein, 1972; Rosenberg, 1977). At the same time, more and more physicians began to specialize (see Table 2.5).

The importance of medical specialization to the quality and cost of the four delivery systems is difficult to overestimate. It is a direct indication of the rapid development of complex and specialized knowledge in medical care. High levels of specialization have led not only to changes in the nature of medical care and the cost of treatment but also to organizational differentiation and the need for coordination.

The trend toward complex or specialized medical care has reached its highest level in the United States, though similar developments have been apparent in each of the other nations, especially Sweden. The pervasive specialization in the United States is even more remarkable considering that as late as 1950 the United States was not particularly exceptional in this regard. In the European systems medical specialization was apparent quite early in the large cities and well-developed hospital systems. Since 1945, European specialization has developed within a context of governmental planning and allocation (albeit to varying degrees), whereas in the United States medical providers themselves have regulated the degree of specialization, flocking to the medical specialties with exceptional speed and making the specialist physician the dominant figure in the medical care delivery system (Stevens, 1966, 1971; Hollingsworth, 1986).

In France, too, medical specialization developed late and rapidly, while midwifery and pharmacy declined sharply and skilled nursing grew relatively slowly. In each of these tendencies the French followed a time pattern similar to that of the United States, but without the extremes in the levels or rates of change observable in the American case. In Great Britain, a rather different pattern is apparent. There, medical specialization jumped immediately after World War II, but since then, it has increased relatively slowly. Moreover, the British system has emphasized the heavy utilization of allied health professionals—as indicated by the continued growth of nursing and midwifery. Sweden, whose somewhat unusual medical system has generated much interest, today resembles the United States more than it does Great Britain in its high degree of physician specialization. Nevertheless, the Swedish system also relies more heavily on skilled nursing and other support personnel than does the American system. As we have seen, the Swedish and American systems differ far more in the nature of state intervention than in the mix of skills and treatment modes available (Stevens, 1966; Berg, 1980).

In specialization as in other respects, different institutional arrangements hold sway in these countries. In contrast to the United States, specialists in France, Great Britain, and Sweden have tended to be concentrated in the hospitals, where historically they have overseen the treatment of patients. General practitioners, who worked on a fee-for-service basis, were generally reluctant to relinquish their patients by sending them to the hospital. In the United States, however, both general practitioners and specialists have usually worked on a fee-for-service basis and have supervised the hospital care of their own patients. Both have had a financial incentive to hospitalize their patients.

In France, the situation has been a bit more complex than in Sweden and Great Britain. For example, in large French hospitals, whether public or private, physicians have been employed on a salaried basis, but in the smaller hospitals—most of them private—physicians have tended to work part-time on the hospital staff and to charge hospital patients for the care they provide. In general, physicians in private practice have not been permitted to care for their patients once they entered public hospitals, where the salaried hospital staff would take over treatment (Rochaix, 1959; Steudler, 1973; Thorsen, 1974; Economic Models, 1976; Bridgman, 1971; Cornillot and Bonamour, 1973; Hatzfeld, 1971; American Medical Association, 1976).

Hospital use, a measure of technological complexity, is tabulated in Table 2.6. In all four countries the hospital has grown in importance as the site for treating patients as the levels of medical technology and specialization have increased, though the timing, rates of change, and levels of hospitalization have varied in the four nations.

Between 1890 and 1970 the United States, despite high levels of medical specialization and medical expenditures, gave less priority to hospital care than did the other three nations. Indeed, while quality has improved, the total per capita supply of hospital beds in the United States has expanded very little since 1940. Throughout the period since 1945, moreover, Americans have had the shortest length of stay in acute-care hospitals, while the Swedes have had the longest. For example, the average length of stay in American hospitals during the early 1980s was 10 days, compared to 24.6 days in Swedish hospitals (Organization for Economic Cooperation and Development, 1985:84).

Great Britain has displayed a similar pattern of little growth in the total number of hospital beds since 1950 and has had virtually no growth in the number of general hospital beds since 1920. Although

Table 2.6. Hospital Beds per 100,000 Population, 1890–1970

Year	United States	Great Britain	France	Sweden
All hospital beds				
1890	NA	628	588	NA
1900	NA	762	659	399
1910	578	882	734	574
1920	767	1,029	754	712
1930	938	1,146	878	922
1940	1,135	1,199	974	1,141
1950	1,212	1,304	1,295	1,249
1960	1,254	1,290	1,489	1,557
1970	1,288	1,335	1,582	1,599
General hospital beds				
1890	NA	365	216	NA
1900	NA	454	245	246
1910	NA	513	269	313
1920	354	559	302	366
1930	367	573	337	467
1940	399	581	367	532
1950	436	570	587	561
1960	461	563	608	661
1970	528	565	656	812

Sources: See Appendix 1.

the patterns are similar, the social conditions responsible for them differ. In the United States, the vast dispersion of population and the market orientation of the system have produced a pattern of few beds per capita in low-density parts of the nation and high levels of competition among hospitals in more densely populated areas. In Great Britain by 1920 there was already a large number of beds per capita and thus a much older stock of hospital facilities in need of constant repair and replacement. Slow economic growth has also constrained the increase in beds, and from 1948 on, the National Health Service has explicitly rationalized the hospital system and rationed the beds.

Like Great Britain, France entered the twentieth century with an extensive and aging stock of hospitals. Until 1940, hospital growth remained quite slow, in part because of substantial resource constraints. In the decades since World War II, however, hospital beds have rapidly increased in number, influenced by many factors, including accelerated economic development, the growth of social insurance funding, and an explicit set of governmental policies (National Center for Health Statistics, 1983). Since 1970, French hospitals have come under strict national planning programs, which govern bed capacity and changes in technology. Even so, the number of beds has continued to grow, and there are great regional inequities in the development of hospitals. Today, approximately 71 percent of hospital costs are financed by social security, 25 percent by private insurance systems, and 4 percent by patients. Under a system implemented in 1984, the French government has resorted to a global budgeting system to limit hospital spending. Under this system, the French government decides how much it will spend on hospital care for the subsequent year, and each hospital is expected to live within its budget. If the hospital runs out of money, however, it can borrow against the next year's budget. Thus far, the plan has succeeded in slowing the rise in hospital spending.

Of the four cases considered here, Sweden is probably the most remarkable for the continuous and rapid growth of its hospital system. In 1890 the Swedish medical system was relatively poor in both physical and human capital endowment compared to the other three nations. Since that time, public policy has pursued expansion in hospital facilities—roughly equally balanced between acute- and chronic-care hospitals. After 1960 this growth slowed somewhat, but the balance shifted to acute care. By 1970 Sweden had more hospital beds per capita—and far more acute-care beds—than any of the other nations (Berg, 1980; Ito, 1980; Serner, 1980).

In general, basic trends in the level of investment in human and physical capital of medical care in the four nations have been similar. In all cases the availability and quality of medical care have improved as medical technology has advanced. These changes have occurred, however, at different rates and at different times. In 1970, as in 1890, each system had a unique mix of characteristics, and throughout the period each system implemented changes in its own distinctive way.

Societal Supply and Demand

Changes in the institutional arrangements of medical systems cannot be understood without attention to the societal environments in which they exist. It is the societal environment that demands certain types of performance, provides the resources to meet these demands, and limits the type of state intervention that may emerge. We might think of these four medical systems as adaptive responses to environmentally created demands under conditions imposed by the resource or supply constraints of the society (Lawrence and Dyer, 1983:86–118; Pfeffer and Salancik, 1978).

Many of the changes in the social, political, and economic structures of Western nations which have had important consequences for medical delivery systems can be captured under three headings: standard of living, demographic transition, and modernization. Increased capacity to pay for medical care, increased need for services among an aging population, and advancements in medical knowledge and technology interact to help shape the demand for and supply of medical services. Taken together, these three trends summarize the forces most influential on the structure and performance of medical systems in France, Sweden, Great Britain, and the United States.

Standard of Living

The standard of living comprises a complex of variables that reflect per capita wealth. Changes in the standard of living influence both the supply of medical care and the demand for it. For example, without significant wealth, it is unlikely that various countries in North America and Western Europe would be allocating approximately 10 percent of their gross national product to personal medical services. During the period between 1890 and 1970, medical knowledge grew exponentially (Price, 1963), nourished by the burgeoning economic growth of Western nations, which made the training, research, equipment, and other necessary facilities possible. Without economic growth, Western medical technology would have been greatly retarded. The rate and the level of economic growth have influenced the timing of changes in the institutional arrangements of medical delivery systems as well as the

types of diseases to which populations have been at risk. For all national medical systems, however they are organized, economic development has been the fundamental prerequisite for medical development.

Economic development, of course, is strongly associated with changes
in the attitudes, expectations, and demographic structure of the population, and these factors we will discuss later. In addition, increases in
the standard of living have greatly modified the nature of medical
needs. Improvements in nutrition and sanitation, for example, which
are directly linked to the rising standard of living, have substantially
reduced the risks of death and disability from infectious diseases, while
immunization and isolation techniques have contributed to this reduction (McKeown, 1976; Powles, 1973). On the negative side, the high
standard of living has risks of death and disability from other causes
(Hollingsworth, 1986; Powles, 1973; Fuchs, 1974, 1986)—for example,
age, sedentary life-styles, overconsumption of food and alcohol, and
environmental pollution.

The single most useful indicator of changes in the standard of living
is the gross national product per capita, corrected for inflation. From
these data, presented in Table 2.7, it is obvious that the growth of per
capita income in France, Britain, Sweden, and the United States has
been dramatic. In 1900 the average of the four nations' real GNP per
capita was approximately $361. By 1970 the average level had in-
creased more than threefold, to $1,371.

There were variations in the pattern of growth. By comparison with
the United States and Great Britain, France and Sweden developed
late, lagging behind through most of the period. After World War II,
however, Sweden and France entered eras of very rapid growth, while
Great Britain and United States grew much more slowly (Denison,
1967, 1974; Williamson, 1974).

Per capita GNP also serves to indicate restrictions on the rate of improvement in medical care, which varied among the four nations. In
this respect the United States has been in the most favorable situation
for system development throughout the period. Until after World War
II, France and Sweden faced greater resource constraints than the
United States. Throughout the entire period, Great Britain had to cope
with growing popular demand for expensive medical technology within
the constraints of a slowly growing economy, even if it started the period at a higher level.

Demographic Transition

The second critical factor in the environment of medical delivery systems involves substantial shifts in the age composition of populations.

Table 2.7. Social Development Components and Index

Year		United States	Great Britain	France	Sweden
1890	GNP[a]	363	500	243	178
	Elderly[b]	3.9	4.5	8.3	7.7
	Education[c]	19.0	8.4	1.2	11.0
	Communication[d]	1	1	1	7
	SDI[e]	.000	.004	.092	.078
1900	GNP	399	510	288	246
	Elderly	4.1	4.7	8.4	8.4
	Education	20.0	9.8	1.8	12.0
	Communication	38	3	5	27
	SDI	.029	.049	.111	.132
1910	GNP	496	521	341	325
	Elderly	4.3	5.2	8.6	8.4
	Education	22.0	11.4	2.5	13.6
	Communication	143	8	7	56
	SDI	.094	.078	.137	.165
1920	GNP	572	451	325	394
	Elderly	4.6	6.0	9.2	8.7
	Education	24.0	12.8	2.9	12.6
	Communication	178	21	9	102
	SDI	.141	.096	.157	.204
1930	GNP	638	507	507	478
	Elderly	5.4	7.4	9.6	9.2
	Education	32.9	14.8	3.4	11.6
	Communication	248	34	20	129
	SDI	.231	.174	.229	.251
1940	GNP	762	599	409	589
	Elderly	6.8	9.2	10.0	10.3
	Education	61.6	19.3	4.4	10.7
	Communication	272	55	29	187
	SDI	.401	.288	.220	.338
1950	GNP	1,029	679	508	821
	Elderly	8.1	10.9	10.3	10.3
	Education	73.1	24.9	6.4	11.5
	Communication	411	76	37	298
	SDI	.590	.397	.267	.432
1960	GNP	1,190	859	730	1,041
	Elderly	9.2	11.8	11.6	11.7
	Education	79.3	29.4	9.0	15.5
	Communication	568	103	84	536
	SDI	.732	.501	.399	.615
1970	GNP	1,555	1,120	1,166	1,641
	Elderly	9.9	12.5	12.1	13.8
	Education	83.9	36.1	13.9	30.0
	Communication	858	192	167	938
	SDI	.943	.641	.574	1,000

Sources: See Appendix 1.

[a]Gross national product per capita in constant 1938 U.S. dollars.
[b]Percentage of population age sixty-five and over.
[c]Secondary-school enrollments as a percentage of population age fifteen to nineteen two decades prior to the date reported.
[d]Annual telephone conversations per capita.
[e]Social development index (for method of construction, see Appendix 2).

One indicator of these changes is the proportion of the population sixty-five or more years of age (see Table 2.7). The size of this age cohort is particularly important in that the type and cost of care needed by this group has presented a major challenge to the capacity of medical delivery systems in recent years.

The effects of aging on the medical delivery systems interacts with the standard of living and the level of medical technology. Many of the important advances in the diagnosis and treatment of diseases and conditions associated with aging are extremely expensive in terms of both personnel and facilities. Moreover, the routine maintenance of the chronically ill aged population has increasingly become professionalized, no longer the province of the extended family. Meantime, as more people have survived to older ages, both the diversity and the average intensity of the medical problems associated with aging have increased. Many illnesses and disabilities would have been fatal before age sixty-five in 1890 now persist into old age, making the treatment problems of the aged not only more complex but more expensive.

The effects of aging on the outputs of medical delivery systems are considerable. For several decades, the proportion of medical expenses generated by the population aged 65 or over have been increasing, and costs far exceed those for any other group. Indeed, the medical needs of the aged are a major factor in the expansion of the costs, facilities, and personnel of medical delivery systems.

Economic development in the West has brought other demographic changes that affect the care of the elderly. With development, populations have moved from rural to urban areas and the extended family has been replaced by nuclear-family patterns. These trends have separated large portions of the population from traditional sources of support in old age or disability. The growth of the welfare state should be seen, in part, as a societal adaptation to the increased economic vulnerability of populations from both aging and economic development (Titmuss, 1958; Easterlin, 1980; Hage, Hanneman, and Gargan, 1989; Flora and Heidenheimer, 1981). In all four countries, the period between 1890 and 1970 witnessed a proliferation of mechanisms for risk sharing through mutual aid, private and public insurance, and direct intervention by governments. These developments in turn profoundly altered the method of decision making in medical delivery systems, resulting in greater centralization under the auspices of the state.

As the data in Table 2.7 demonstrate, the populations of these four nations have aged at various rates and with quite different timing. Great Britain and the United States had relatively young populations at the end of the nineteenth century, reflecting the population growth attendant upon early industrialization (and, in the United States, high rates of immigration). France and Sweden, on the other hand, had a larger percentage of aged citizens, consistent with slower population growth. Even though the proportions of the elderly populations in France and Sweden were roughly the same at the turn of the century, however, the causes were quite different. Acting on the ideals of equality expressed in the French Revolution, Napoleon had abolished primogeniture, which was a custom in large parts of France. All children were to share equally in the division of property—amounts of which tended to be quite small (Le Roy Ladurie, 1974). It was the very small plots of land which limited the number of children in families. As birth rates dropped, the proportion of the elderly in the population increased. In Sweden, by contrast, the aging of the population was due partly to various public health measures, partly to the generally better health of a rural population in the nineteenth century, and partly to the out-migration of younger people to the United States during the late nineteenth century. Gradually, however, the four nations have converged as birth rates have declined in the United States and Great Britain and the average length of life has increased.

As we have suggested, the differences in age structure are somewhat related to the amount of state intervention. For example, the countries whose governments were highly involved in the delivery of medical services early on also had sizable percentages of citizens sixty-five and over. This is not to suggest that the age structure was the most important cause for state involvement in the delivery of medical services, but increases in the proportion of the elderly have generated pressures on the state to provide medical as well as other social services for them.

How important the age factor is for state intervention is illustrated in the case of France. Starting in 1890, half the days of hospitalization were attributable to the elderly. Whereas the average length of stay for an acute-care patient was 36 days, the average for an elderly patient was 229 days. The French had already created an elaborate system of hospices, or hospitals for the elderly (Rochaix, 1959), at the beginning of the nineteenth century. And for the next fifty years, more than half of the hospital patient-days were devoted to care of the elderly (Rochaix, 1959:191). Thus, the sizable elderly population in France at the turn of the century is one reason why the public sector began to intervene early. And historically the relatively small elderly population in the United States is an important reason why the Americans were so late in adopting some form of public financial care for the elderly.

Modernization

As economies develop, people's attitudes and expectations about health change, transforming the mix of consumer demands for medical care, which affect the structure of medical delivery systems. It is useful to differentiate between the "need" and the "effective demand" for medical care. The need for specific types of care is related to levels of health, as well as the age of a population, standard of living, and the technological capacity of the medical delivery system. Effective demand comprises need but also requires that those in need have some awareness of their need, formulate a desire for medical intervention, and have access to resources to pay for it. In the process of translating need into demand, the population's belief in the efficacy of medical intervention is extremely important. We have attempted to capture this aspect of demand formation at the aggregate level by examining trends in the levels of formal education and communication (see Table 2.7).

Of course, levels of formal education and communication are rather indirect indicators of beliefs, attitudes, and expectations about medical care. Unfortunately, more direct evidence, such as survey research, is unavailable in all countries throughout the period. In any case, even if the indicators are indirect, it is clear that popular attitudes toward medical care in each of the four nations have changed over time in such a way as to increase demand. For example, in 1890, the vast majority of people in all four nations viewed physicians with suspicion and avoided hospitalization whenever possible (Abel-Smith, 1964; Hollingsworth, 1986; Rosenberg, 1987; Starr, 1982; Heidenheimer and Elvander, 1980). By 1980, however, the public believed so strongly in the efficacy of physicians and hospitals that many analysts believed that medical care professionals and facilities were overutilized (Enthovan, 1980; Olson, 1981; Starr, 1982).

In some respects, the massive shift in public attitudes is easy to understand, in that some contemporary medical technology is demonstrably more efficacious than that practiced in 1890 (Starr, 1982; Stevens, 1971). It is important to note, however, that changes in perceptions about the efficaciousness of medical technology were facilitated by changes in the educational and communications systems of these four countries. Educational development was especially important. Schools served as "transmission belts" for the ideology of science in general and scientific medicine in particular. They were also directly used in public health campaigns (for immunization, sanitation, dietary habits, fluoridation, etc.), and in some countries, educational authorities increasingly brought the young into contact with the medical delivery system via school medical services and health inspectors (Political and Economic Planning, 1937; Gilbert, 1966; McCleary, 1933). The expanding volume of mass communication in Western societies also contributed to the diffusion of changing beliefs about the efficacy of scientific medicine. Not only did the quality of medical care change markedly during the period between 1890 and 1970, but members of Western societies were increasingly "bombarded" with testimonials to the wonders of medical technology.

Let us ignore for the moment whether the demand for medical services is in the public or private sector. It is significant that the timing and the extent of the demand for medical services have differed substantially in these four nations. The data presented in Table 2.7 on levels of education and communication must serve as proxies for direct measures of the demand for medical care, which are virtually unobtainable. This table demonstrates the relatively early beginning and rapid diffusion of secondary education in the United States, as well as the later, less extensive development in Sweden and Great Britain, and the late expansion of popular secondary education in France (Prost, 1988; Peterson, 1952; Hage, Hanneman, and Gargan, 1989; Archer, 1982; Ringer, 1979; Husen, 1969a and b; Flora, 1983; Walters and Rubinson, 1983; Garnier and Hout, 1981; Stone, 1976; Meyer et al., 1979).

The volume of communication per capita in the United States was generally higher than that in the other nations, partly because we have chosen telephone usage as the indicator. This technology developed first and diffused more rapidly in the United States. Telephone usage is also related to the greater per capita real wealth and greater population dispersion in the United States, which may have accelerated the diffusion of this medium of communication. In all four countries, as the level of education increased and communication systems expanded, citizens became increasingly aware of changes in medical technology and demanded access to it. This demand in turn fostered more advances in medical technology.

The substantial variations in levels of education and communication and the timing of their development, treated as proxies for the demand for medical services, indicate how the nature of demand has varied among the four countries. It appears that the American case was somewhat more exceptional after 1920, and Sweden displayed unusually rapid development, commencing shortly after World War II. France and Great Britain lagged as late as 1970. Throughout the period, Americans have been exceptional in both proxy indicators of the diffusion of knowledge about (ergo demand for) medical technology.

If we hypothesize that the differential rates of development in these medical systems were driven by changes in technology and the economic resources of the society, the situation of the United States was the most favorable over the entire time period. Between 1890 and the end of World War II, both the level and rate of economic and social development in the United States were somewhat higher than in the other three nations. Furthermore, throughout the period, the population of the United States was substantially younger than that of the other three countries. This factor was very much responsible for the different patterns of growth in the four medical delivery systems. The European nations (especially Sweden and France) were forced to confront the problems of old age and chronic illness much earlier than the United States. Taken together, social, economic, and demographic factors—the overall social environment—produced a medical delivery system in the United States different from those evolving in the three other cases. In Table 2.7 these factors are summarized in a single index (the social development index) to be used in later analyses.

France and Sweden in many respects had similar social, economic, and demographic bases for the development of medical delivery systems. In 1890 both nations were poorer, less well educated, and had substantially older populations than the United States. Both countries were predominantly agricultural. Throughout the period between 1890 and 1950, however, France and Sweden experienced considerable social and economic development, though both countries still diverged substantially from the United States. After World War II, however, economic and social development surged. Sweden, especially, underwent what can only be called spectacular social and economic transformation (Stephens, 1979; Korpi, 1978, 1983).

At the turn of the century, Great Britain was in a rather favorable position for rapid medical system development, with high levels of per capita income, a fairly well developed educational and communication system, and a relatively young population. Except for the quick aging of the population, however, social development in Britain was extremely slow and nearly linear compared to the other nations.

The levels, timing, and composition of change in the social environment of the medical systems of the four nations suggest substantial diversity in both the qualitative and quantitative constraints and opportunities for the expansion of medical care. And the expansion and development of state intervention in the medical delivery systems in these four nations reflect, in part, this diversity.

Social Development and Patterns of Institutional Evolution

In this chapter in addition to outlining the major variables in this research, we want to describe the relationship between social development and the evolving institutional arrangements of the medical systems of France, Great Britain, Sweden, and the United States between 1890 and 1970. We cannot pretend to analyze the histories of these systems in all their complexity. Rather, we focus on a few critical variables. By examining variations in the investment in human capital, the level of specialization, and the degree of state intervention, it has been possible to sketch the similarities and differences in the histories of these systems.

In all four nations the demand for medical care has mushroomed. Between 1900 and 1980 the share of gross national product devoted directly to personal medical services tripled or quadrupled, the number of academically trained physicians per capita increased substantially, the supply of hospital beds per capita at least doubled in three of the four nations (Great Britain being the exception), and the degree of specialization among physicians rose dramatically. These substantial increases in the size and complexity of the medical care delivery systems have created a need for reorganization, rationalization, and coordination. In all four nations, despite marked divergences in the nature and extent of intervention, the state has played a leading role in the coordination of medical services.

Even though the same basic forces have been at work in France, Great Britain, Sweden, and the United States, the evolutionary pattern of each system has been unique. The medical systems of the four nations were very different in 1890, have made different policy choices since then, and have differed in the timing of their changes and in the level of their capacity. As a result, the four systems display substantial variation in structure and performance in the contemporary period.

By 1970 the medical care delivery system of the United States was the most expensive, most specialized, and least governmentally coordinated of the four cases. This pattern resulted from a variety of forces: early and rapid economic development and modernization, the large size of the system, and a strong tradition of a weak state. Throughout the period from 1890 to 1970 the private sector attempted to meet the rising demand for medical care. During the 1960s and 1970s, however, a slower rate of economic growth, together with the pressures of an aging population and more demand for equal access to and greater integration and rationalization of the medical system, brought the first tentative steps toward centralized state coordination.

The British, too, entered the twentieth century with a predominantly private medical care delivery system, but during the period the system changed comprehensively. The slower economic growth and stronger traditions of governmental intervention in Britain gave rise to an early and widespread reform of the medical delivery system. By 1970 the National Health Service had become a rather extensive system of bureaucratic medicine (Hollingsworth, 1986).

France and Sweden have displayed many similarities but have diverged nevertheless. Both entered the twentieth century with long traditions of state coordination of certain aspects of their medical systems, and economic development came late to both. Sweden moved rapidly toward an expensive, specialized, hospital-based system—and did so almost entirely through explicit policy choices in a system in which the state was a major actor. The French system grew more slowly and preserved a "mixed" approach, combining state intervention and the marketplace.

Each of the four exceedingly complex systems has adapted to differing challenges in varying ways. We have sought to depict at least the flavor of this diversity, though by no means can a short chapter do justice to it. To augment the general picture we have drawn, path analysis of the relationships among the key variables—social development, number of doctors, level of specialization, and state intervention—may prove useful.

In the decades between 1890 and 1970, most Western societies experienced substantial improvements in the quality of medical care and health. Life expectancy grew along with social development and profound changes in the structure and technology of medical delivery systems. In recent years, scholars have debated the causes of improved health and longevity, some attributing these to a rising standard of living, others to medical technology. One body of literature has minimized the importance of "modern medicine" in reducing death rates during the twentieth century (McKeown, 1976a and b; McKeown and Record, 1962). We believe, however, that changes in the standard of living and in the medical care of Western societies are intertwined. A more proper question to ask is how social development has affected the institutional arrangements of medical systems. Social development was in many ways a necessary precondition for the development of twentieth-century medical systems, and in some respects twentieth-century medical knowledge has influenced the course of social development. We offer two hypotheses:

2.1. net of other factors, the higher the level of social development, the greater the level of human-capital investment in medical delivery systems.

2.2. net of other factors, the higher the level of social development, the greater the degree of state intervention in the delivery of medical services.

Zero-order correlation coefficients essentially confirm these statements. The correlations between social development and the human-capital/medical-complexity variables are $\geq.79$. To be sensitive to the interplay of demand, supply, and intervention variables, however, we have used recursive path analyses to provide more complex explanations.

The path analysis diagram in Figure 2.1 proposes that the demand variables represented by the social development index are exogenous to such medical delivery system characteristics as the number of physicians and the level of technological complexity (the proportion of physicians who are specialists). The characteristics of these medical systems, however, are very much influenced by the level of social development, as well as various random factors. The level of revenue derived from the central government is a response of the combined effects of the level of social development and human capital/medical complexity. The degree of centralized state control over prices and personnel is represented as causally subsequent to central control over revenues, the supply variables, and the level of social development.

This path analysis, though not a precise specification of the dynamics of the growth in medical expenditures, is a relatively accurate ordering of the variables, as subsequent discussion will show (Stevens, 1966, 1971; Steudler, 1973; Heidenheimer and Elvander, 1980; Hollingsworth and Hanneman, 1984; Hollingsworth, 1986). Moreover, the estimates of the path coefficients in Figure 2.1 suggest a rather interesting story about the dynamics of the development of institutional arrangements. With path analysis, we are able to examine the direct and indirect effects of independent variables on dependent variables. Thus, in Figure 2.1 we can assess how social development has directly influenced human capital and state intervention. We can also assess how social development indirectly affected state-intervention variables through human-capital variables. Finally, we can understand how demand (social development), human capital, and state control over revenues affect state control over prices and personnel. This type of statistical analysis, combined with our other historical investigations, allow us to reach several conclusions about the institutional development of national medical systems, especially their choice of administrative form, one of the more interesting aspects of institutional analysis. Why do some countries choose a system in the private sector and others accept various forms of state intervention? In fact, the systems in these four countries have all evolved toward greater and greater state intervention, as we have demonstrated. Here our concern is with a brief and more formal analysis of the choice of institutional arrangements.

Although path analysis allows us to disentangle the complex sequence of events, especially when there are time-series data, there are some problems with relying too heavily on it. We believe it is important not to reify path coefficients but instead to understand their social and institutional context through study of both qualitative and quantitative

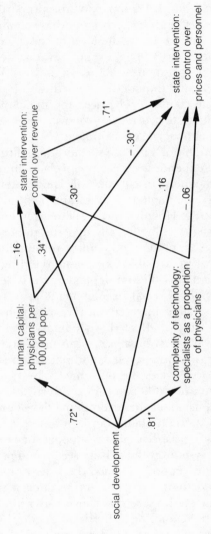

human capital: physicians per 100,000 pop.

state intervention: control over revenue

state intervention: control over prices and personnel

social development

complexity of technology: specialists as a proportion of physicians

.72*

.81*

−.16

.34*

.30*

.16

−.06

.71*

−.30*

Note: Standardized partial regression coefficients by the Parks GLS method are shown on paths.

*p < .05, one-tailed; N = 36.

Figure 2.1. Social Development and Institutional Arrangements: Empirical Results

data. Too often, moreover, those who employ path analysis misinterpret the causal processes underlying the path diagram. There is a tendency to perceive a single cause and then to impute this as the major force. But societies are not so simple. Typically, complex causal networks underpin each of the paths employed in an analysis (Hage and Meeker, 1988). With these ideas in mind, we now wish to sketch some of the causal processes that connect the growth in social development, as we have measured it, and the investment in human capital.

Social Development and Investment in Human Capital

It is perhaps reasonable to assume that increases in social development reflect a growth in demand, and to some extent, we share this perspective, as later discussion will demonstrate. For now it is sufficient to note that the demand for medical care increases with income level, aging of the population, education, and improvements in communication. Better education and societal communication expand awareness about both preventive medicine and modern medical technologies. But the extremely high path coefficient of .72 between social development and the density of physicians and the even larger coefficient of .81 between social development and the proportion of specialists among physicians cannot be accounted for by a simple increase in demand.

A second, less obvious explanation for the link among these variables is the growth in knowledge about medical care. Between 1890 and 1970 a great deal of specialized scientific research provided the foundation for much of the progress in medical care (later, we will return to the debate about the effects of biomedical knowledge on mortality). For example, work in the biological sciences by Louis Pasteur in France and Robert Koch in Germany allowed the development of vaccines (to be discussed in detail later). Similarly, the discovery of anesthesia brought improvements in surgery, and the discovery of x-rays advanced diagnosis and treatment. Scientific instruments such as the cytoscope, the rectoscope, and the bronchoscope enabled doctors to learn more about human physiology.

Since these developments at the turn of the century, laboratory tests have grown more varied and sophisticated. Equipment such as the electron microscope has permitted major breakthroughs in biological research. New technologies for diagnosis and treatment have emerged, including open-heart surgery, the CAT scanner, kidney dialysis, and organ transplants. Less technologically complicated but nonetheless powerful treatments involve new medications, including penicillin and other antibiotics, antidepressants, anticoagulants, etc.—all of which have transformed the practice of medicine.

As societal wealth has grown, willingness to invest in scientific research, especially on the human body, has also increased. Researchers who widen the boundaries of medical knowledge require and have received considerable funding. Their research has resulted in complex and expensive technology and new forms of diagnosis and treatment. These developments have fostered an increase in ancillary or paramedical personnel and greater specialization of doctors.

The key point here is that there would be little demand unless there were new technologies and treatment. It has been the growth in knowledge which has given doctors more opportunities to improve patient care and which has justified the increases in the number of physicians per 100,000 population. This is not to deny the barrier that expensive treatments have erected for populations with limited financial resources. Nevertheless, it is clear that *increased belief* in the efficacy of medical care has contributed to the demand for that care and has affected the institutional arrangements of medical delivery systems both directly and indirectly. Irrespective of the objective reality about the efficacy of medical technology in the twentieth century, increased faith in the capacity of medical technology to prevent, cure, or ameliorate illness has influenced the rapid expansion in the volume of medical treatments and the support for investments in research, human capital, and medical specialization. Not only did the citizens of these four countries have more resources available to pay for medical treatment in 1970 than they did in 1890, but they were willing to spend a larger share.

Choice of Institutional Arrangements

Social development affects state intervention in the domains of revenue and control over prices and personnel differently. These differences reveal a great deal about why some aspects of medical systems diffuse and some do not.

The coefficient of .34 between social development and state control over medical revenues indicates that during the past century as societies have become wealthier and better educated, and their populations have aged and become more aware of changing medical technology, there has been a considerable shift toward more state funding of medical care. Most of these societies started with some form of private insurance—typically for workers, as in the friendly societies in Great Britain or the mutual aid societies in France—often augmented by public assistance as well as private charity. These institutional arrangements could not cope with the burgeoning costs of medical care, especially hospitals, and so the state in each of these four countries has become increasingly involved in funding more expensive care for various populations and in equalizing access to care.

We must qualify these observations, however. First, the extent of state intervention in the funding of medical care has varied in these four countries. Second, the timing of intervention was different in each country and was related to diverse historical events and traditions. In general, the state first moved to support medical care for workers and veterans (Orloff and Skocpol, 1984; Hollingsworth, 1986). As these programs expanded to cover dependents, the state became substantially involved in funding. Only the United States, by concentrating on compensatory programs such as Medicaid and Medicare, has lagged far behind the other three countries.

Changing public attitudes toward medical technology also affected the way medical systems were coordinated and integrated. Recognizing that "good health" is a highly salient political issue, political parties, labor unions, and other groups have attempted to redefine access to medical care as a "right" of their members (Wilensky et al., 1985). The growth of third-party payment, whether under state or private auspices, is partially a consequence of increasing popular demand for access to medical care.

In those nations where political parties have given high priority to health issues or where the provision of medical care has historically been of considerable governmental concern, access to medical care has been explicitly recognized as a right to be guaranteed by government (Hollingsworth and Hanneman, 1984; Heidenheimer and Elvander, 1980). Thus, increasing bureaucratization and state involvement were, in part, responses to changing public attitudes about medical technology. Variations in organized interest groups, however, have differentiated attitudes toward how the structure of medical delivery systems should be organized in different countries (Hollingsworth, 1986; Hollingsworth and Hanneman, 1984). Where the working class was racially or ethnically fragmented (for example, the United States), it had less ability to mobilize politically, and the demand for public, centralized medical facilities was relatively slow to develop. Likewise, France was slow to develop a social security system largely because of ideological and political splits in its working class, which allowed only low levels of mobilization, as in the United States (Stephens, 1979). Furthermore, the strong French state has been much more resistant than some to class pressures (Wilensky, 1976; Hage et al., 1989). On the other hand, in more ethnically homogeneous societies like the Swedish and the British, the working class has been better able to mobilize political power and to capture control of leftist political parties. In Britain and in

Sweden, in contrast to the United States, there has been a high degree of state intervention (Hollingsworth, 1986).

State funding of medical care is not the decisive institutional arrangement in shaping the costs and social efficiency of national medical systems, however. More critical is the extent to which the state attempts to control prices and personnel, as we demonstrate in the following chapters. In this respect, institutional arrangements do not necessarily diffuse well, contrary to what some of the diffusion literature would have us believe (DiMaggio and Powell, 1983). For example, the path coefficient between social development and state control over prices and personnel is only .16. There is no uniform and inevitable movement toward state regulation of medical costs. In one sense, state coordination of medical costs tends to reflect two different stages in the development of national medical systems. Citizens and their elected representatives become concerned first about access to services and only later about their costs. This process also reflects a long-term tendency for the working class to shift toward middle-class "consciousness," becoming more concerned about cost containment and less concerned about access issues.

It is our observation that the state becomes involved in the control of prices and personnel only slowly. In the face of much opposition from the medical profession, for example, the French state edged toward effective control of physician fees. In general, states are reluctant to encounter the opposition of the powerful medical profession (Hollingsworth, 1986; Starr, 1983). Yet the incentive to intervene grows as the costs of medical care escalate. Slowly, even the American state is beginning to make serious efforts to control costs.

But there are countervailing forces as well. It is true that the number of doctors has a strong influence on state intervention. Historically, doctors have been a powerful interest group and have often fought against state control of medical revenues ($\beta = -.16$) and especially state control of prices and personnel ($\beta = -.30$). The proportion of specialists has had a positive effect on state intervention, however. Indeed, the sum of the indirect and direct effects of specialists on state control over prices and personnel has been positive.

The reasons for this relationship are complex. In Europe and, to a lesser extent, in the United States, specialists historically have tended to be concentrated in hospitals. State control has often meant control over hospital prices and personnel. The higher educated and more specialized physicians associated with the hospital have tended to accept hospital controls over personnel and, indirectly, state coordination through state oversight of hospitals. Until 1970, specialists, especially in

Europe, tended to benefit from such intervention (Hollingsworth, 1986; Abel-Smith, 1965). Thus, specialization (and the technological complexity that accompanies it) seems to be positively related to the type and quantity of state intervention.

Our analysis thus far leads to a very important insight about the consequences of investing in human capital, that is, training physicians and medical personnel. Societal investment in human capital has subsidized a profession with its own interests. If doctors are able to halt the movement of the state toward price regulation, there may be certain consequences, consequences that are considered in later chapters.

To comprehend why some societies have a great deal of state intervention and some very little, we must also understand the growth in the medical profession and its timing, the mobilization of the industrial working class and other consumer groups that pressure the state to provide health care, and finally the strength of the state. Although these interactions are worthy of another book, here we can briefly indicate that where the state has been strong and the working class has been well mobilized but the medical profession did not become powerful or active until after the mobilization of the working class, the state intervened early. Where the state has been weak, the working class not well mobilized, and the medical profession relatively powerful prior to the mobilization of the working class, then state intervention has been more modest. Sweden and Great Britain were closer to the first paradigm, whereas France and the United States were closer to the second. Moreover, within the second paradigm, the French have had a stronger state than the Americans, and the American medical profession has been more powerful vis-à-vis the state and the working class than was the case historically in France (Hollingsworth, 1986).

On the basis of previous empirical work (Hollingsworth and Hanneman, 1984), we have observed that several dimensions of state intervention are highly correlated, though the degree of centralized state control over revenue often has been quite different from the level of state involvement in control over prices and personnel. In Figure 2.1, the path coefficient between these two variables is .71. In subsequent chapters, we are concerned with how the performance of the four medical delivery systems has been influenced by two different dimensions of state intervention: first, the degree of centralized state control over medical revenues, and second, a combined index that measures the degree of centralized state control over prices of medical services and appointment of medical personnel.

How decisions about the delivery of medical services are made, resources are allocated, and activities are coordinated very much influence the performance of delivery systems—as the remainder of this book will demonstrate. Each country has attempted to modify the performance of its medical systems through various types of policies. In succeeding chapters we attempt to demonstrate how system performance has been influenced by the degree of state intervention as well as investments in human capital.

3

THE COSTS OF CARE

Between 1890 and 1970, the proportion of the gross national product devoted to personal medical services increased dramatically in all Western nations. For several decades spending on medical care has been growing more rapidly than the gross national product in all four countries of concern here. In the United States and a few other Western countries, the cost of medical care now exceeds 10 percent of the gross national product, more than the amount spent on national defense or education, two other major institutional sectors of society. Only pensions and social security assume a larger share of the total value of goods and services produced per year. Moreover, despite the many efforts at containment, costs continue to rise. The United States and those few Western European countries that still have relatively young populations can expect considerable upward pressure on medical costs as their populations age. The reasons for this growth and strategies for containing it have become major issues for policy analysts and major sources of concern for the state.

Several cross-national studies have focused on the costs of medical care (Maxwell, 1981; International Labor Office, 1959; Abel-Smith, 1963, 1967; Simanis, 1973; Organization for Economic Cooperation and Development, 1977). But unlike ours, previous studies have not discussed the development of several national systems over a long period. Ours is the first systematic effort to estimate medical expenditures throughout the twentieth century. Data on medical expenditures prior to 1929 have been rare and have usually delineated only public expenditures. In contrast, our investigation is based on all public and private expenditures for personal medical services.

By our best estimates, per capita expenditures for personal medical services (in constant 1938 United States dollars) increased sevenfold in England and Wales between 1900 and 1971, ninefold in France from 1891 to 1971, forty-six times in Sweden, and fourteen times in the United States. The largest part of these increases occurred following World War II.

Most Western countries have attempted to control costs through specific policies, but they have generally been relatively unsuccessful, for most governmental policies have not been designed to alter the basic institutional arrangements of the medical delivery system. We maintain that the underlying structural arrangement of a medical delivery system shapes performance. If the state makes mere incremental changes without directly intervening to control prices, personnel, and other parts of the medical system which influence costs, the results are likely to be negligible.

Microeconomics has dominated the thinking about medical cost control, especially in the United States. The argument for the privatization of medical care is a plea for competition, under the assumption that the medical sector operates similarly to the home construction industry— that is, that the same laws of supply and demand apply. Since this is such a common assumption in much of current discussion about privatization, it would be well to address it here. We propose to discuss how supply and demand operate at the microlevel in the medical arena, presenting evidence to show that they operate in a fashion essentially opposite to what microeconomic theory would predict. To complement the discussion of a privatized perspective, we also introduce a theoretical discussion about how state mechanisms of coordination and control function to contain costs.

The first section of this chapter specifies the determinants of the demand and supply for medical care. Next, we compare market mechanisms of coordination to those of the state. Because the discussion is relatively abstract, we provide concrete details about how the state in each of the four countries intervenes to control costs. We explore the sharp contrast between the United States, with its preference for private-sector coordination, and the European countries, with various types of state coordination. With this background in place, we give a quantitative analysis of our findings for Britain, France, Sweden and the United States during the period between 1890 and 1970.

Determinants of Medical Costs

The Demand for Medical Care

We have suggested that as the level of social development increases, so does the level of medical expenditure. To measure social development we devised an index combining gross national product, levels of education and communication (that is, modernization), and a measure of demographic structure. Each of these components helps to shape the demand for medical care, which influences costs.

Several studies have demonstrated that as the wealth of countries rises so does their spending on medical care. In the terminology of economics, medical care is a luxury rather than a necessity, and a characteristic of luxuries is that at some point in the economic development of a society, their consumption tends to increase at a faster rate than income (Jonsson, 1981; Newhouse, 1978). Consequently, at some point in their development countries tend to begin increasing the share of GNP devoted to medical care.

The history of medicine suggests that as medical technology advances, it creates more work for itself. As more of the young survive to advanced ages, more of the population suffers chronic diseases, which are difficult and expensive—if not impossible—to cure. Because the desire for and the possibilities of greater knowledge are unlimited, the resources demanded for medical services continue to increase. Thus, once a society can afford basic necessities, it tends to spend increasing amounts on medical care. Because there is no proper way to evaluate need, the insatiable demand for more simply escalates exponentially as the resources of the society expand. A nation can have the medical care that it can afford or is willing to pay for (Maxwell, 1981:9–11; Seale, 1959).

A second set of demands for medical care has resulted from increases in the levels of formal education and communication, or the degree of modernization, which has expanded awareness of modern medical treatment and belief in its efficacy. Many studies have demonstrated that the more educated consumers become, the more they are aware of their medical needs and the more initiative they will assume in demanding medical care. Ronald Andersen, Bjorn Smedby, and Odin W. Anderson in their surveys of populations in Sweden and the United States (1970) correlated educational level with frequency of physician visits and use of other medical services. Myron J. Lefcowitz (1973) demonstrated with American data that after controlling for age, education was more important than income in influencing the use of medical services. These studies suggest that the more educated an individual, the greater the likelihood that the person will be exposed to and influenced by health information. As the level of education rises, the individual becomes more alert to information about health (Grossman, 1972, 1976; Fuchs, 1986), is more likely to accept the claims of modern medicine, and tends to use more medical services (Lefcowitz, 1973; Donabedian, 1976). Although the prices of medical services are largely shaped by providers, the costs nevertheless are somewhat influenced by consumer demand.

Under some circumstances, education may reduce the demand for medical services and thus potentially reduce costs as well. Part of the medical information the public absorbs has to do with preventive medicine. The interest in jogging and exercise, the concern about weight, the elimination or reduction in smoking and drinking, the consumption of more healthful foods, the campaign against teenage drinking, etc., obviously represent a potentially powerful impact on the incidence of illness and accidents. In other words, preventive medicine has the potential to reduce medical costs (Grossman, 1972, 1976; Russell, 1986). Education may also encourage early intervention that prevents more serious disease and helps reduce costs. Certain diagnostic tests can reveal the early stages of hypertension or other diseases and forestall the more serious consequences that might ensue if the early indications went unnoticed. We will return to this point when we discuss the differences in medical care and mortality rates by social class.

As medical technology expands, communication spreads information about its alleged effects throughout the society. The nature of the communication system in a given time and place helps determine how much information a population receives about the nature of the medical services available to it. The more extensive the information, the greater the demand for medical care. In short, increases in education and communication provide people with more information about medical technology, encouraging more use of medical facilities and higher expenditures for medical services. But again, increased communication can also disseminate information that improves health, reduces mortality, and lowers costs as a consequence (Russell, 1986). Some newspapers in the United States—the *Washington Post*, the *New York Times*, the *Los Angeles Times*, for example—have regular columns on health care each week, and the National Cancer Institute and other such organizations work to educate the public, too.

As the standard of living rises in societies, the proportion of the population age sixty-five and over tends to increase. Deaths in childbirth and from infectious diseases have been greatly reduced. In their place, cardiac and pulmonary disease, cancer, and a variety of chronic conditions have become the leading causes of death. The technologies available for treating the new mix of conditions are not curative but are highly expensive. In other words, as populations age, they become more susceptible to neoplastic and degenerative diseases—many of which are expensive to treat. Therefore, medical expenditures increase as the proportion of the population sixty-five and older rises. Taking Britain as an example, approximately 13 percent of the population in 1970 was over age sixty-five, but this group occupied 48 percent of general hospital beds and 44 percent of psychiatric beds (Maxwell, 1981:89). In Sweden at about the same time, approximately 10 percent of the population was over age seventy, but this group used about half of all hospital bed-days, and those over eighty made up only 2.5 percent of the population but used 25 percent of all hospital care (Jonsson, 1981).

Though all these demand variables are exogenous to the medical delivery system, they do substantially influence the level of spending in medical care. Nevertheless, even when these variables are taken together, they do not account for all the variation over time and across countries in the level of medical spending. So far these factors appear to function very much as an economist would predict. Demographic, economic, and other variables specify the demand function. Apparently, the level of education of the society, the nature of its communication system, and the society's demographic structure largely shape demand. But this perception is somewhat misleading. Everyone wants quality health care, and the measure of quality is subject to infinite modification. The medical sector is much different from the automobile or the clothing sector, where demand has much clearer limits. Perhaps these differences will become clearer as we shift to the problem of supply.

Supply Considerations

In our analysis, there are essentially two supply variables: the number of physicians and the proportion of physicians who are specialists. According to neoclassical economic theory, marketplaces—including the medical world—tend to operate alike according to the laws of supply and demand. Neoclassicists would therefore predict that increasing the number of physicians would raise the quantity of medical services and lower their price (Newhouse, 1978). There is not much empirical evidence to support such a view, however. Indeed, the empirical evidence supports the opposite view (Fuchs, 1986:chap. 4). The theoretical explanation is that medical services are not competitive in the same way the housing market is competitive. Physicians have considerable ability to induce demand for their services, and increasing the number of physicians tends to create more work, thus driving up medical costs (Newhouse, 1978:56; Evans, 1974; Lewis, 1969; Fuchs, 1986).

We may take the level of specialization among physicians as a proxy for advances in medical technology. A medical delivery system, once it attains a certain level of technology, tends to strive for even more complex levels. Medical specialization, a surrogate for medical technology, is difficult to contain, for specialization has an inherent dynamic: it has an appetite for learning, and knowledge tends to be self-generating. Specialization demands new occupations and new capital equipment (Hage and Aiken, 1970; Stevens, 1971). The more specialized the medical delivery system, the greater the number of complex diagnostic tests and treatments that can be performed on patients, thus escalating costs (Aaron and Schwartz, 1984).

The physician is the major actor in this process. Even if professional fees constitute a decreasing percentage of the total medical bill, the physician determines the type and quantity of medical treatment. It is the physician who prescribes drugs, decides the length of hospital stay, recommends surgery or other procedures, arranges for x-rays and other diagnostic tests. The physician, as Victor Fuchs (1974b) points out, "is the gatekeeper to the production of medical care."

Among physicians, specialists are especially prone to raise costs. Many studies demonstrate that specialists charge higher fees, order more (and more complicated and costly) tests, and hospitalize more patients (Blackstone, 1977; Donabedian, 1976; Davis, 1974). We certainly do not mean to suggest that specialists are primarily motivated by a desire to maximize their income. Much evidence suggests that specialists are largely concerned with the best interests of their patients and the winning of their patients' approval (Feldstein, 1970; Fein, 1967; Donabedian, 1976). Nevertheless, specialists have a tendency to do everything they have been trained to do, regardless of the cost-benefit ratio, and the more training they have, the more likely they are to pursue every option (Fuchs, 1986, 1974b). In addition, specialists tend to use whatever facilities are at their command. Several studies have demonstrated that the notion of allocating medical technology based on a medical assessment of need has little meaning. The perception of need simply tends to grow in response to provision, for specialists react to an expansion of supply by redefining need along a continuum (Cooper, 1974). Instead of meeting a preexisting, relatively stable level of demand, increasing the number of doctors and specialists simply increases the demand for care and the costs of services (Donabedian, 1976; Feldstein, 1967; Fuchs, 1986).

Market versus State Coordination

We have discussed the major forces pushing delivery systems in the direction of increasing medical costs, but the effects of societal development and expanding medical technology on system performance also depend on another factor: how decisions are made and activities coordinated within the medical care delivery system. We have suggested that the coordination of treatment decisions by providers and consumers without external supervision is likely to lead to a *socially* inefficient allocation of resources. This hypothesis must be examined more closely, and an alternative model—coordination by state "hierarchy"—compared to it.

Classical economic theory holds that in a perfect market, prices are minimized, productivity is maximized, and the amount and distribution of transactions are optimally efficient. Adam Smith coined the phrase "the invisible hand" as a way of thinking about the guiding forces of the market place. More recently economists and others have theorized that under some circumstances the visible hand of management can achieve lower prices and better distribution than the marketplace (Williamson, 1975, 1985; Chandler, 1977). To understand the conditions under which coordination by hierarchy or the visible hand of management is effective in maximizing social efficiency, we must unearth some of the assumptions buried in the theory of the markeplace.

The achievement of optimal efficiency by market coordination depends on certain factors: there must be large numbers of producers and consumers; each producer and consumer must behave in a cost-minimizing, profit-maximizing fashion; and each producer and consumer must have a high level of knowledge about the products and market conditions. Distortion may be introduced into the behavior of markets if the commodity is very expensive (involving high levels of investment to produce substantial levels of saving to the purchaser), is an "indivisible" commodity (such as clean air or, to a lesser degree, a hospital), or the technology is so complex that consumers cannot assess their need for it or its quality. The notion of a "perfect" market is, of course, an ideal type.

Many transactions occur with reasonable social efficiency even in the presence of considerable market imperfections, but market coordination of the production and consumption of medical care creates a situation that may raise health care costs. For the marketplace to perform as Adam Smith predicted, consumers must be well informed and able to choose among alternatives, but a vast literature (see especially Donabedian, 1976) demonstrates that consumers have inadequate knowledge about the quality of medical services. As George Monsma (1970) has argued, many, probably most, consumers cannot judge the quality of physicians or the relative advantages of one course of treatment over another. One major study (Trussell, Morehead, and Erlich, 1961) showed that almost all patients believed they were getting quality medical care, yet few were, according to medical educators who examined the medical charts. About 50 percent of the hysterectomies, for example, were considered unnecessary. Perhaps the most striking finding was the differential quality of care practiced by physicians with the same level of training—board certification—in different kinds of hospitals. Thus a major prerequisite—that consumers be well informed—does not appear to be satisfied in the medical sector.

The difficulty of evaluating quality and price is compounded by the fact that medical care is not a single standardized product but a whole series of "products." There are many kinds of illnesses, each demanding different treatments, for instance. Then too, a portion of the cost of modern medical care systems is devoted simply to connecting the patient with the appropriate specialized service. At the level of highly specialized treatment, moreover, patients rarely have the ability to choose alternative providers. Nor does increasing the supply of physicians reduce costs. Instead, the greater the number of physicians in a particular locality, the higher the fee charged per visit. In addition, physicians in the United States typically receive higher fees for admissions to the hospital than for patient visits. Thus, even though services cost more in the hospital setting than in the office or in a patient's home, American physicians have had a financial incentive to hospitalize their patients. Research also shows that the greater the number of hospitals in a particular area, the greater the number of services duplicated in each hospital and therefore the higher the cost per patient (Hollingsworth and Hollingsworth, 1987).

What causes hospitals to duplicate expensive technology? Physicians, especially specialists, want the latest technologies. Many in the United States are affiliated with several hospitals, and they tend to send their patients to those with the newest technologies. The competition for patients among hospitals thus provides physicians with a considerable degree of power and hospital administrators with a considerable incentive to obtain the technologies requested by the physicians. Having the latest equipment and the most complex technologies lends prestige that gives a hospital an advantage in the competition for both physicians and patients. Many hospitals want to practice the well-publicized procedures, such as open-heart surgery and heart transplants. Perhaps the CAT scanner is the best example of expensive equipment that is duplicated in many American hospitals, where a competitive environment has driven the demand for costly technology.

In the place of coordination by the market, alternative institutions for allocating and coordinating resources have emerged. In most nations various mechanisms often originated at the local level. For example, in the United States, physicians have increasingly been drawn into clinic and hospital-based practice rather than remain as solo practitioners in the private office. Medical associations, professional societies, and professional review committees constrain the behavior of both providers and consumers in medical care. More and more medical decisions in the United States are made outside a "free market," as insurance plans and contractual arrangements between physicians and consumer groups shape the delivery of medical services. At the national level, massive fiscal and administrative interventions by the state have entirely removed many allocational decisions from the market, thus replacing "market" coordination with a state "hierarchical" coordination system.

If "privatized" systems become less socially efficient in allocating medical resources as levels of specialization rise, we must, of course, ask whether state intervention may be expected to do any better. We do not maintain that state coordination produces universally and uniformly "better" medical care, but there are several reasons to expect that it can reduce costs, especially for highly specialized, technologically sophisticated services. Clearly, certain forms of state coordination substantially constrain spending.

As in the case of the market, there are ideal types of state coordination. In the most centralized form of state coordination, a single decision-making authority controls the entire process of production (that is, the supply and qualifications of providers; the numbers, types, and locations of facilities; access to facilities; the price of services) and distribution (which patients receive which treatments; who pays the bill). In principle, this type of state coordination removes many of the barriers to optimal allocation present in market-oriented systems. Centralization makes more complete information available to decision makers, enabling them to plan the supply and location of human and physical capital resources so as to reduce duplication of services and to assure the provision of at least minimum services to all areas. That is, the delivery of medical services may be managed in such a way as to reduce the dual tendencies of "overproduction" and "underconsumption" inherent in imperfect medical markets. Because control as well as information is centralized, such systems tend to have greater capacity to implement change and to plan long-range development than do market-based systems.

In general, a system in which the state pays for many of the services but imposes few limits on their consumption, distribution, and prices tends to drive up the costs and consumption of services. Fortunately, the four countries involved in this study provide considerable variation in the way in which revenues, prices, and personnel have been coordinated for an extended period of time.

Theoretically, the state is not the only agent that could effectively control revenue, prices, and personnel in the medical sector. Indeed, the health maintenance organizations that proliferated in the United States during the 1970s and 1980s were designed to control the costs of medical care by exercising greater control over prices and personnel. A single HMO, from which all medical revenues were derived and which set all prices for medical services and appointed all medical personnel, might be as effective in controlling medical spending as a centralized government regulator. In practice, of course, any existing HMO or similar private organization is likely to control only a modest portion of revenues, prices, and personnel. The competition among HMOs is likely to lead not only to a higher quality of medical service but also to higher costs than those that would exist under a single central authority.

Hierarchical systems realize certain economies of scale. Some of the information costs inherent in actors' attempts at rationality in an imperfect market are eliminated, for their choices are restricted and decisions are made for them. Substantial economies of scale may be realized by higher utilization of fewer high-cost facilities (especially specialists and hospitals) and the reduction or elimination of duplication. Expensive equipment, such as CAT scanners, can be allocated regionally on the basis of need. Similarly, one or two hospitals in a metropolitan area can be designated to handle all the difficult but rarer illnesses.

Systems characterized by a high degree of centralization under state auspices may also produce more socially efficient outcomes in a different way. Where the decisions about the allocation of resources for medical care are made by a small number of authorities (as in hierarchies), rather than by large numbers of individuals (as in markets), powerful provider groups have less influence in shaping allocation. In market-oriented systems, physicians have more power than state administrators in allocating resources. In systems with substantial state coordination, the administrators or state bureaucrats can more easily resist pressure from providers. Of course, on a day-to-day basis, providers may have considerable autonomy in the use of what resources have been delegated to them by state authorities. In general, state-coordinated systems try to control costs by distributing resources to provide general services for the entire population. Usually, though not always, medical policies that improve the lives of many people—even if very slightly—are more "socially efficient" than policy choices that improve the lives of few people—even if very greatly. And this is one of the major differences between market-oriented and state-oriented systems. The state-dominated system provides few resources for the highly specialized needs of the few. Such people—if they have the resources—will receive better and more expensive care in the market-oriented system, even if it is less socially efficient.

The tendency for state-coordinated systems to make allocational decisions that minimize medical costs, comes from two sources. First, state coordination overcomes some of the delay and the defects in information dissemination inherent in markets characterized by highly specialized and high-cost services. Second, decision makers in hierarchical systems are subject to influence by mass participation and are likely to pursue policies that benefit larger numbers of persons, rather than fewer. On balance, such programs are more likely to promote the general health of the population.

Thus, the state is able to reduce costs through several mechanisms. The first and most critical is the avoidance of equipment duplication. The second is the achievement of economies of scale by aggregating low-frequency, high-cost cases in specially designated hospitals. The third and perhaps most obvious is direct control of prices, which is the basis of our measure of state intervention. In sum, we maintain not that only state intervention can effectively control revenue, prices, and personnel but that variation in the degree of centralized state coordination of medical revenue, prices, and personnel influences variation in medical costs.

Our research is designed to assess the degree to which state intervention affects medical expenditures. To that end, we want to focus on two polar systems, those of the United States and Great Britain. At one end of the continuum, the United States historically has had the most privatized medical delivery system and has been least effective in controlling escalating medical expenditures. At the other end, the British system—especially since 1948, when the National Health Service came into existence—has been the most centralized coordinating system and has had the most capacity to constrain the escalation. The French and the Swedish systems have fallen between the extremes of the National Health Service and the American system.

The American System

From various tables in Chapter 2, it is apparent that as late as 1970 centralized controls over revenue, personnel, and prices were substantially lower in the United States than in the other three countries. Prior to World War II, medical technology in the United States, as in most other countries, was relatively simple, but during and after the war it became much more complex (Stevens, 1971, 1989; Hollingsworth, 1986; Hollingsworth and Hollingsworth, 1987). In response to escalating complexity and cost, medical insurance, financed for the most part in the private sector, became increasingly prevalent. And as third-party coverage became more widespread, the American population tended to use more physician and hospital services and to spend more on medical care. Then during the 1960s, state and central governments took over funding a large proportion of medical services with the introduction of Medicare and Medicaid (Marmor, 1973; Hollingsworth, 1986; Starr, 1982).

A system in which third-party coverage pays on a fee-for-service basis is generally more expensive than a capitation-payment system, and in the United States the third-party retrospective system of reimbursing medical expenditures substantially eliminated fiscal constraints on providers and consumers. By 1970 the elderly and the indigent were covered by Medicare and Medicaid, and a high percentage of other Americans had some form of medical insurance. By its very nature, the reimbursement system gave patients, physicians, and hospitals little incentive to consider costs when making decisions about medical care. Rather, the system encouraged more costly types of care. Though physicians were the gatekeepers to medical care, most physicians by 1970 had little knowledge about the costs of care and had incentives not to be concerned (Enthoven, 1980:xvii, 212). The structure of the system encouraged the use of medical technology all along the line, and quality was the doctor's wild card and the provider's defense against proposals for change (McNerney, 1980). In contrast to earlier periods in the twentieth century, the well-trained physician was increasingly able to practice without having to worry about the ability of patients to pay their medical bills.

Similarly, American hospitals had few incentives to take costs into account or to make consumption and production choices. American hospitals competed with one another not by reducing costs, which, it was assumed, insurers would pay, but by trying to outdo one another in the scope and technological complexity of services. For example, when one hospital acquired a CAT scanner, neighboring hospitals attempted to acquire the same technology, even if the area needed, in terms of economies of scale, only one CAT scanner.

The American retrospective system of payment rewarded behavior that increased costs and punished behavior that attempted to contain costs. American hospitals were reimbursed on the basis of either costs or charges based on costs, and more costs meant more revenue for the hospitals, for most costs were passed on to third-party payers. Obviously, such a system proved to be somewhat inflationary and wasteful (Enthoven, 1978, 1980:xvii), and Americans spent an increasing percentage of the gross national product on medical care.

For several years following its inception, federal funding for Medicare and Medicaid was relatively open-ended. The range of services was broad, and the cost-based reimbursement system encouraged providers to dispense unnecessary services and to raise their fees. Moreover, public funding—like other third-party payment schemes—encouraged patients to use more services than would otherwise have been the case. In short, an open-ended funding system threatened to produce open-ended spending on medical care (Mead, 1977:40–41; Enthoven, 1980).

Although medical costs dramatically increased once Medicare and Medicaid came into existence, it was, of course, not only these programs but the structure of the entire system which drove up medical costs. Even the American system of taxation contributed. Following the 1940s, the tax system provided a major subsidy for the purchase of health insurance, by allowing employers to deduct the cost of employees' health insurance as a business expense. At the same time this benefit was not considered income taxable to employees and was not included in the base on which social security taxes were computed. Medical benefit packages became a by-product of the collective bargaining process in the United States, although such arrangements were not necessarily the most efficient way of using medical dollars. Martin Feldstein and Bernard Friedman (1977) have estimated that on the margin, the tax subsidy represented approximately 35 percent of the cost of health insurance (Meyer, 1981). The tax laws also encouraged employers and employees to buy medical insurance with low deductibles, so that most medical bills could be paid with untaxed rather than after-tax dollars. Elsewhere, Feldstein (1973) estimated that most wage earners were able to purchase nearly 50 percent more medical care for the same money in this fashion. Most consumers had little incentive to question the value of medical service or to seek out less costly care (Enthoven, 1980).

Over time, providers of medical care in the United States justified their opposition to state cost-control efforts by invoking the sanctity of the doctor-patient relationship, arguing that it was improper for groups other than the organized profession to monitor professional decisions. Certainly physicians may be sincere in wishing to protect the doctor-patient relationship, but as the state paid an increasing proportion of the nation's medical bill, it had a vested interest in controlling costs. Even so, the power of the American medical providers severely limited the options for effective controls (Hollingsworth, 1986).

Historically, the American medical delivery system has been very competitive, but as we have seen, markets do not function in the medical sector to control spending. As this anomaly began to be recognized during the 1960s and 1970s, state and federal governments began resorting to a variety of regulatory devices to control medical spending. We believe that cost controls are likely to be effective only if there is state coordination of the price of medical goods and services and the appointment of personnel, but this kind of coordination would require a fundamental restructuring of the American medical system. Instead, the Americans kept the existing institutional arrangements intact and tried modest regulatory devices. One study after another has found this kind of government regulation relatively ineffectual in curbing the costs of medical care (Joskow, 1980; Steinwald and Sloan, 1980).

One basic problem with the American strategy to control medical costs through regulation is the sheer difficulty of regulating the medical industry. Public regulation is more effective in those industries in which there are few providers, a single product, and very good information on the efficaciousness of the technology. None of these criteria applies to the field of medicine. Instead of few providers, there were in the United States in the 1950s and 1960s more than six thousand hospitals and several hundred thousand physicians, a large proportion of whom were in private practice. Instead of a single or a simple product, medicine has numerous products, and even highly qualified practitioners often disagree about treatment strategy. Industries in which there are trade-offs among competing values are especially difficult to regulate. For example, the decision between kidney dialysis and a transplant for a patient with renal failure is difficult to make purely on the basis of statistics.

The Americans have thus had a competitive medical system in which they have relied on privatized coordination dominated by provider interests and somewhat regulated by the state. Without any mechanism for coordinating revenues, prices, and personnel, the system had little capacity to control medical expenditures.

The British System

Throughout much of the twentieth century Great Britain has had lower levels of income, education, and communication—all on a per capita basis—than the United States. Within the medical delivery system, Britain has had fewer physicians per capita too and a smaller proportion of specialists. With the variables generating demand for medical services lower in Britain than in the United States, one would expect medical expenditures to be somewhat lower. At the same time, medical care has long been more accessible in Britain, under a system that exempts a large proportion of consumers from the direct responsibility to pay for medical services. This kind of "free" care would have driven up the demand for medical care and the costs were it not that Britain for some years has had effective state controls over revenue, prices, and personnel (Hollingsworth and Hanneman, 1983; Hollingsworth, 1986; Stevens, 1966; Klein, 1983).

Throughout the twentieth century, local and central governments in Britain have been much more involved in the appointment of personnel than in the United States. Partly for this reason, the medical profession in Britain has exercised less autonomy in shaping the costs of the system. Prior to 1929, approximately one-sixth of the nation's doctors were employed by the state as district medical officers, charged with administering Poor Law medical relief. By 1948, when the National Health Service came into existence, virtually all doctors were employed by the state, though those who worked in the hospital were employed under a different system from that employing those who worked outside. In both cases, the state controlled the number of practitioners. A doctor could go to work in a hospital under the National Health Service only when there was an opening, and the number of openings was controlled by the state, which had nationalized all hospitals in 1948. When an opening did occur in a hospital, the regional hospital board appointed a doctor, who might then practice in a number of different hospitals in the region. The general practitioner had somewhat more autonomy about where to set up shop, but the government designated certain places as over-doctored, and general practitioners were expected to avoid these. Administratively, general practitioners who worked within the National Health Service were appointed by local executive councils (Stevens, 1966; Hollingsworth, 1986).

In Britain, administrative decisions about the medical system and decisions about medical treatments have been much more concentrated than in the United States. Prior to 1948, the state used a very complex procedure to make administrative decisions about the number of patients per doctor, expenditures per patient, and expenditures per doctor. For example, in 1912 when the National Health Insurance program began, the costs per patient and per physician were primarily a public decision determined by the state. After the creation of the National Health Service, Parliament in theory approved expenditures, and between 1948 and 1974, the local executive councils and the regional hospital boards received from the central government the previous year's budget plus a small increase. The system provided relatively effective centralized controls over spending decisions.

The effect of state controls over revenues and expenditures is reflected in the acquisition of new capital equipment under the National

Health Service, and it is also in this area that the consequences of rationing were often most controversial. Until 1970 the restrictions on capital expenditures in the National Health Service—including those for hospitals—were considerable. Money and building materials in postwar Britain were in short supply, and priority was given to the construction of houses and schools. Of course, capital investment could not be permanently postponed if the quality of medical services was to be maintained. The desirable level of capital investment in a national health delivery system depends on many considerations—the quality of the existing equipment, the speed with which technology is changing, the ability of the existing system to accommodate the demand for care. Whatever the criteria, however, the National Health Service, in its early years, spent relatively little money on capital investment. For example, during the first six years of the National Health Service, less than 1 percent of all national investment was allocated to capital investment in the medical sector (Abel-Smith and Titmuss, 1956).

It is impossible to estimate the level of capital expenditure that would have been invested in hospital construction had there been no National Health Service, but the ratio of capital expenditures on hospitals to all expenditures on hospitals was far lower than it had been before World War II and far less than the United States was spending in the early 1950s. Capital expenditures represented 19.6 percent of all expenditures in 1938–1939 but only 4.1 percent in the early 1950s, while the Americans were spending 23.4 percent of their hospital budget on hospital construction (Abel-Smith and Titmus, 1956:133–36).

Because of variability in hospital design and usage, there are no reliable data on the maximum lifespan of a hospital. In general, hospitals in twentieth-century Western Europe and North America have lasted only twenty-five to forty years. At that rate of replacement, well over half the hospitals in the United Kingdom would have been replaced by 1975. It should not be assumed, however, that simply because a building is old, it is unsatisfactory. The Americans, who are more accustomed to having the latest technology, have had a tendency to replace hospitals, but the British, being less wealthy and more concerned with costs, have been more likely to adapt, upgrade and extend hospital structures.

The French and Swedish Systems

In degree of state intervention the French and Swedish systems have fallen between the British and American poles since World War II. Before the war Sweden had more state coordination than any of the other three systems, and its relatively high level of state intervention since the war years is a legacy of this involvement. Historically, the Swedish state had long played an important role in the delivery of medical services. Because Sweden lagged behind in industrialization and because its population was relatively dispersed in rural areas, it lacked the concentrated populations necessary to sustain a sizable private medical practice. And because there was no large private medical pratice, the Swedish Medical Association was late in developing and has never been very strong politically (Ito, 1980; Anderson, 1972). Indeed, as early as 1920 approximately 60 percent of all physicians were employed by the state (Ito, 1980). Because Swedish doctors were poorly organized and because Sweden was a relatively poor country, medical technology was not well developed before World War II, and medical expenditures were low relative to the other three countries.

By the end of the war, however, Sweden was industrializing rapidly and becoming more prosperous. While the medical profession remained relatively weak politically, consumers were better organized and more politically powerful than in the other three countries. They were demanding a modern medical system, and in a relatively short period of time, they were able to achieve their goals. Sweden now has one of the most modern medical delivery systems.

But the central government in Sweden has been less involved than the British in revenue collection and the ownership of facilities. Whereas in Britain the central state provided much of the revenue for the National Health Service, in Sweden the county councils provided approximately 75 percent of medical expenses. Funding for hospitals was derived primarily from the counties and major municipalities, and the central government contributed very little to capital improvements (Anderson, 1972; Sidel and Sidel, 1977). Prior to 1970, ambulatory care in Sweden was provided neither by a capitation system nor generally by salaried providers as in Britain but on a payment-per-visit basis. Swedish patients had many more options as to where to enter the system than their British counterparts. They could consult a general practitioner or voluntarily enter a hospital outpatient department. Moreover, the Swedish state did not exercise the same degree of control over medical specialization as did the British government (Heidenheimer and Elvander, 1980). Partly as a result, patients tended to gravitate to the most expensive centers for outpatient care. For example, in Britain, a very high proportion of outpatient care was provided by general practitioners, but by 1970 at least half of Sweden's outpatient care was provided by hospital-based doctors (Berg, 1980:41).

Since World War II Sweden's high medical costs have largely been due to a relatively high GNP, a large elderly population, and a widespread societal demand for specialization and technology unexcelled anywhere (Heidenheimer and Elvander, 1980). But part of the costs were due to rather ineffective state controls over medical prices and personnel. Sweden did make a serious effort to avoid the duplication of expensive services and to rationalize the costs of medical care, but the counties could not control costs as effectively as the more centralized state system of Britain. As a result, between 1950 and the latter part of the 1970s, the per capita expenditures on personal health services increased in Britain by approximately 500 percent, but in Sweden, the increase was 2,500 percent (Anderson and Bjorkman, 1980:228).

The structure of the French medical delivery system since 1945 resembled the American more than the British or Swedish. In France there were both public and nonprofit hospitals, most physicians were in private practice, and most physician services were paid on a fee-for-service basis. In France too, as in the United States, most of the medical services financed by the state have been provided in the private sector. The two systems differ in the scope of state financing, however. In the United States, coverage is limited primarily to the indigent and the aged, whereas in France, coverage is more universal and fees and prices are effectively controlled by the state. Until recently, the French system, unlike the British, exercised little control over the number of specialists and where physicians might practice (Willoughby, 1966; Cornillot and Bonamour, 1973; Bridgman, 1971; Thorsen, 1974; Economic Models, 1976).

Before 1960, French physicians essentially determined their own fees, and the patient paid the doctor. The patient then presented the receipt for payment to the social security fund, which reimbursed a portion of the charges. Beginning in 1960 (Hatzfeld, 1971), the state set maximum fees for different services after negotiating with various physicians' associations. To discourage overuse of medical services, fees were not to be refunded in full. For example, routine physicians services were reimbursed at 80 percent following the payment of an initial deductible, specialist payments were reimbursed at 70 percent, and 80 to 100 percent of hospital costs were reimbursed (Thorsen, 1974:50). As a disincentive, patients consulting doctors who did not subscribe to the government's fee schedule were reimbursed at very low levels (usually 20 to 40 percent of the cost of care). The overall result was to bring at least 95 percent of all physicians under the government's fee-setting scheme (Thorsen, 1974:53; Economic Models, 1976:vii). Because the patient paid a deductible and a portion of the bill, the government exercised less centralized control over revenues than in Britian. Neverthless, the deductible and coinsurance, combined with state control over fees, did restrain escalating costs.

Medical Costs

The dependent variable in this section of the chapter is medical expenditures in constant prices. Because we are concerned only with personal medical services, we have excluded such collective goods as expenditures for water supply, sewage, and clean air—even though these clearly have beneficial effects on health. Moreover, we have excluded expenditures called "sickness insurance," when these have been used for income maintenance.

The estimation of our time series on medical expenditures was exceedingly complex. For each country, we had fairly reliable data on medical expenditures for recent decades, but for the earlier period we estimated expenditures from a variety of sources, which are discussed in Appendix 1. Appendix 3 contains a discussion of the strengths and weaknesses of our quantitative methods.

In analyzing the data for this chapter, we found the logarithmic transformation of medical expenditure a more appropriate test of our hypotheses than an equation that uses only the original score for each observation. This finding indicates that the relationship among state intervention, human capital investment, social development, and other variables, on the one hand, and medical expenditures per capita, on the other, are often nonlinear and of a "diminishing returns" type. That is, a change of one unit in state intervention at a low level produces a larger unit change in the dependent variable than a change of one unit in intervention at a higher level. Where such nonlinearities better fit the data in either the standardized partial regression coefficient or path analytic models shown in the next section, this difference of interpretation is of substantive interest.

We have suggested that both demand and supply increase medical costs, whereas state intervention will reduce them. In Table 3.1, we present quantitative data relevant to these hypotheses. The direct effects shown in the table, which are standardized partial regression coefficients, permit us to examine the direct effects of demand, supply, and state intervention variables on medical expenditures, one at a time. The coefficients are consistent with our hypotheses. The effect of centralized state control over revenues is substantial and positive, while centralized state control over prices and personnel has substantial cost-constraining effect, once the other variables are held constant. The relationship between the demand variable—social development—and medical expenditures is strong, but the relationships between the supply variables and costs are weaker. To put these relationships in other

Table 3.1. Decomposition of Effects of Social Development and Delivery System Variables on Log Real Medical Expenditures per Capita

State intervention: price and personnel control	
Direct effect	−.58
Net causal effects	−.58
State intervention: revenue control	
Direct effect	+.37
Via state price and personnel control	−.41
Net causal effects	−.04
Physicians per 100,000 population	
Direct effect	+.18
Via state intervention	+.18
Net causal effects	+.36
Specialists as proportion of physicians	
Direct effect	+.29
Via state intervention	+.02
Net causal effects	+.31
Social development	
Direct effect	+.33
Via state intervention alone	−.10
Via medical system variables alone	+.36
Via medical system and state intervention	+.16
Net causal effects	+.75

Note: Table is based on the model in Figure 3.1. The effects reported for each independent variable are defined as follows: the "direct effect of X on Y" is equal to the standardized partial regression coefficient of Y on X, controlling for the other variables shown; the "effects of X on Y via Z" is defined as the sum of all indirect effects connecting X and Y which pass through Z as the last mediating variable in the chain (in some cases, there may be several such effects).

GLS zero-order regression coefficients with log real medical expenditure (* is significant at .05, one-tail): price and personnel control −.11; revenue control +.44*; physicians per population +.76*; specialists as proportion of physicians +.73*; social development +.79*.

terms, once social demand variables are taken into account, human capital and medical complexity do have direct effects on costs. Yet, given supply-and-demand considerations, state intervention also makes a cost difference. State intervention via revenue drives costs up, but state control of prices and personnel reduces costs.

The results displayed in Table 3.1 strongly suggest that the sources of medical expenditures are indeed multifaceted. Although the "demand-pull" view is supported by these results, it is also important to note that the effects of the institutional arrangements of the medical system on medical expenditures are substantial and in good part independent of demand.

One of the most interesting findings is the confirmation of the bivalent effects of state attempts to impose bureaucratic forms of organization on medical delivery systems. As anticipated, state subsidization of medical costs without accompanying control over prices and the allocation of personnel tends to contribute to cost expansion. Equally important, yet often misinterpreted because of its historical association with state provision of revenue, state controls over prices and personnel appear to exert a substantial constraining effect on medical expenditures.

Having found support for our main hypotheses about the effects of the structure of the delivery system on medical expenditures, we next examine these relationships in a different, somewhat more speculative manner in order to enhance our understanding of the process by which delivery system structures influence medical costs. We present in Figure 3.1 a recursive path model of how social development, the human capital variables, and centralization under the auspices of the state influence medical expenditures. This model permits us to move beyond the direct effects, just discussed, to assess the indirect effects of demand and supply variables as they are mediated through state intervention variables. We can assess the indirect effects, by examining the net causal effects entries in Table 3.1.

A decomposition of the effects of this model provides interesting insight into the process by which medical expenditures have increased. The effects of social development on medical spending, both direct (+.33) and indirect, are strong and positive. The direct effect of physician supply on medical expenditures (+.18) is further evidence that the medical profession plays some role in increasing medical expenditures. But much of the effect of provider supply on medical expenditures are mediated via greater state intervention. The coefficients indicate that the more physicians, the less control exercised by centralized governments and the greater the expenditures for medical care. These data suggest, first, that the more numerous the physicians, the more influence they exert against state intervention, and second, that the weaker the control of the state, the higher the level of medical expenditures.

The development of specialization among physicians, with its attendant bias toward hospital-centered capital-intensive technologies, appears from the decomposition in Table 3.1 to have relatively small effects on costs. The direct effect is indeed positive (+.29), but the indirect effects explain virtually none of the variation in medical expenditures among the four countries through the period.

From a theoretical point of view, the most interesting data in Table 3.1 relate to the effects of state intervention on medical expenditures. Many analysts have assumed that since increasing governmental involvement in medical delivery system activities has historically coincided with rapidly increasing costs, more centralized controls must be a major cause of rising levels of medical expenditures. The decomposition of the model, however, suggests that this has not been the case.

True, the direct effect of increased state involvement in the financ-

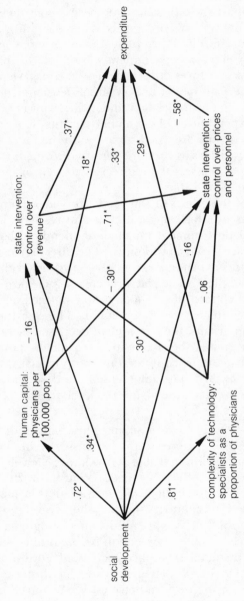

Note: Standardized partial regression coefficients by the Parks GLS method are shown on paths.

*p < .05, one-tailed; N = 36.

Figure 3.1. Effects of Social Development and Delivery System Variables on Log Real Medical Expenditures per Capita

ing of medical care, net of all other influences, has been to increase medical expenditures (+.37). In these four cases, however, increasing state involvement in the financing of medical care has tended to bring about greater control by the state over medical prices and personnel, sometimes coincident with financial involvement, but more often subsequently (Hollingsworth and Hanneman, 1983; Hollingsworth, 1986). Increasing centralized state control of prices and personnel has tended to offset the greater costs due to greater state collection of revenues for medical care. In fact, the substantial combined impact of state centralization over the control of medical revenues, personnel, and prices on medical expenditures offsets much of the effects of physician supply and specialization on medical expenditures.

The data in this chapter clearly suggest that private-sector forms of coordination are relatively ineffective in controlling medical expenditures, compared to state coordination. Although state financing tends to increase medical expenditures, centralized state control over pricing and personnel tends to contain the growth of these expenditures.

Certain policy implications of this chapter merit close consideration. The effect of demographic, attitudinal, and wealth variables on the cost of medical care may diminish in future years but is unlikely to reverse. In any event, these forces are largely beyond the immediate control of policy makers. On the basis of our data analysis, it appears that strategies to limit the number of medical professionals and to deemphasize medical specialization could exert some downward pressure on the total cost of medical care. Without state controls over prices, however, the consequences of limiting the number of professionals and the level of specialization are likely to be very modest. Although state control over revenues may be necessary for cost containment, it has not historically been sufficient. Thus, it appears that among the various strategies available to policy makers, one of the best suited to cost containment under conditions of heavy demand pressure in highly complex and specialized medical delivery systems is centralized state control over prices and personnel. The adoption of such a policy would be difficult in some countries, for it would require a fundamental change in the historically derived institutional arrangements. Nevertheless, the logic of a privatized system tends to produce duplication of medical services and an upward spiral of costs, which the state has some capacity to contain.

4

IMPROVING LEVELS OF HEALTH

By any measure, the health of populations in Europe and North America improved markedly in the years between 1890 and 1970. Life expectancy increased substantially and age-sex standardized mortality rates declined by 50 percent, while infant, neonatal, and maternal mortality rates fell even more rapidly. Disability due to illness became less prevalent, and levels of height and overall physical well-being of populations increased. About these conclusions there is little disagreement.

About the causes of these improvements in health, however, there has been much debate. Most analysts agree that rapidly rising standards of living, better and more universal education, and basic public health measures (sewage and water treatment, pest control, vaccinations, etc.) have played a major part. More controversial are the roles played by advances in biomedical knowledge, medical therapy, and the organizational structure of medical delivery systems. Some analysts are skeptical of claims that changes in medical technology and the delivery of medical services have been responsible for any significant improvement in levels of health (McKeown, 1975, 1976a, 1976b; McKeown and Record, 1962; McKeown, Record, and Turner, 1975; McKinlay and McKinlay, 1977; Powles, 1973). A few have maintained that much of modern medical practice is actually counterproductive (Illich, 1976). Thus far, however, few writers have explored exactly how levels of health are influenced by changes in biomedical knowledge and the organizational structure of medical delivery systems.

In this chapter, we attempt to provide some insights into the causes and processes underlying the improvement of health in Britain, France, Sweden, and the United States since 1890. We cannot, of course, offer definitive answers, but we hope to shed some light by confronting this issue in a somewhat unusual way. Rather than ask whether changes in the standard of living *or* biomedical knowledge and technology *or* the organizational structure of medical delivery systems are primarily responsible for improvements in levels of health, we prefer to explore how all these changes interact.

We hypothesize that biomedical knowledge and technology and the organizational structure of medical delivery systems have contributed to changes in the overall level of health during the past century in two ways: first and more obvious, the structure has determined how specific new types of preventive, curative, and palliative treatments have been delivered to various populations; second, the structure has affected the way in which the standard of living, the level of education, and the age-sex population distribution (that is, societal development) influence levels of health. For example, the extent to which increases in the standard of living give rise to improved levels of health depends on whether new knowledge emerges, how that knowledge is diffused, and therefore how medical delivery systems are organized.

Heretofore, we have distinguished the organizational structure of medical delivery systems along two dimensions: the number and specialization of physicians and the degree of state coordination. As a means of organizing our discussion of the effects of the structure of medical delivery systems on the overall health of society, this distinction remains useful.

Human Capital Investment and the Level of Health

Despite arguments to the contrary, it seems clear that the dramatic increases in the resources allocated to the development of medical knowledge and technology since 1890 are strongly connected to the improving general health of Western societies. The advances in knowledge about immunization, nutrition, sanitation, as well as the diagnosis and the treatment of specific diseases have substantially reduced mortality. Obviously, biomedical knowledge is not limited to a curative model. Indeed, many of its most important contributions have related to preventive medicine. And the medical profession has been important in diffusing new knowledge about health to the general population. But the effectiveness of the medical profession in disseminating information has been influenced by the institutional structure of the medical delivery system. Taking these arguments together, we can hypothesize that

4.1. net of other factors, the higher the density of providers, the wider the diffusion of knowledge about health throughout the society and the higher the level of population health, and

4.2. net of other factors, the higher the density of providers, the greater the allocation of societal resources to medical care and hence the higher the level of population health.

The hypothesis that increasing the number of providers per capita (that is, density of providers) improves societal health, *net of other factors,* presents the simple argument that at any given level of societal development, biomedical knowledge, and system integration, an increase in the number of providers leads to better diffusion of knowledge related to health and medical care, and these in turn improve access and so improve levels of health.

In several widely acclaimed studies, Thomas McKeown and his colleagues (McKeown, 1976a, 1976b; McKeown, Record, and Turner, 1975; McKeown and Record, 1962) have argued that much of the observed improvement in societal health in the Western nations occurred for reasons other than the growth of scientific medicine and medical therapy. There is much to be said in favor of McKeown's arguments (and we shall return to them later in this chapter), but it is important to recognize that the role of biomedical knowledge and technology was not limited to immunization and medical therapies. Biomedical knowledge, diffused through the medical profession, also led to the monitoring and isolation of infectious diseases; public health efforts against disease vectors; general environmental health measures such as water purification, sewage treatment, factory safety, and safe food processing procedures; and improved nutrition and cleanliness. It was groups within the modern medical establishment that disseminated much information about diet and "healthful behavior," just as they have initiated and supported health education programs throughout the past century (Woods and Woodward, 1984; Smith, 1979; Novak, 1973; Richards and Woodward, 1984). For all these reasons, we believe that much of the influence of social development (for example, increases in levels of wealth and education and improvements in communication) on population health is properly seen as being mediated by simultaneous changes in biomedical knowledge and in the organizational structure of medical delivery systems.

4.3. We hypothesize that the indirect effect of social development on health, as mediated by investment in human capital, is greater than the direct effect. A major point of this hypothesis is that physicians and other medical providers are technological gatekeepers for the health system. They influence not only the delivery of medical services but public health policy as well. Indeed, most public health officials responsible for sanitation, disease control, and immunization have traditionally been physicians. In other words, much biomedical knowledge has been disseminated *via* public health systems. (On the complexity of this subject, see Novak, 1973; Brand, 1961, 1965; Macleod, 1967; Richards and Woodward, 1984; Wohl, 1983; Riley, 1986; Apple, 1987; Tarr and McMichael, 1977).

Nevertheless, the effect of physicians and the medical establishment on societal health has not been entirely salutary. As medical care has become more complex, specialized, fragmented, and differentiated, the problems of assuring access and coordinating the delivery of medical services have become very difficult. In each of the four nations we are considering, most physicians before World War II—and many since then—tended to favor market and voluntary associational forms of organization to cope with the problem of coordination. Opposition of organized physicians and the medical industry to state intervention was a pronounced theme in the histories of France, Great Britain, and the United States during most of the first half of this century, though the nature, strength, and effectiveness of this opposition varied greatly from country to country (Hollingsworth, 1986; Stevens, 1966, 1971; Macleod, 1967; Heidenheimer and Elvander, 1980; Eckstein, 1958). There are, of course, many ways of coordinating the delivery of medical services other than by the intervention of the state, but coordinative efforts by states have tended, primarily for political reasons, to emphasize egalitarian access to demonstrably efficacious technologies. From this line of argument, we hypothesize that

4.4. net of other factors, the higher the density of providers, the lower the level of governmental coordination of medical service delivery and hence the lower the level of population health.

Increasing the number of physicians has both positive and negative effects on population health. On the positive side, as the quantity of medical services—both public and private—has increased, societies have acquired more information about how to improve levels of health. On the other hand, insofar as medical practitioners have impeded the development of state coordination, and thus better access to medical services, they have slowed the rate of improvement in the general health of the population.

Specialization also has an effect on population health. We hypothesize that

4.5. net of other factors, the greater the level of specialization, the greater the level of population health;

4.6. net of other factors, the higher the level of specialization and the more societal resources allocated to medical care, the higher the level of population health; and

4.7. net of other factors, the higher the level of specialization, the less state coordination of medical services and hence the less access to medical services and the lower the level of population health.

The rationale for these hypotheses is similar but not identical to our hypotheses about the numbers of physicians. The idea that increases in the level of specialization contribute directly to increases in population health is based on the view that the increases in medical knowledge and technological complexity associated with specialization improve the efficacy of medical interventions. Some of the effects of specialization on population health act in common with increased expenditures on medical care. A portion of the historical association between increasing societal development and improved levels of health is due to advances in and diffusion of biomedical knowledge (4.3).

Extensive specialization in a nation may also act to limit the degree of state coordination and thus slow the rate of improvement in population health. This last effect arises from two sources. First, specialization in medical practice indicates a well-developed medical establishment capable of defending its interests through economic and political influence. In a number of Western countries—especially before World War II—the ideological position of organized medical practitioners was generally opposed to state coordination (Stevens, 1966, 1971; Novak, 1973; Hollingsworth, 1986). Second, as we have already discussed, organizational systems that are highly differentiated and specialized tend, all other things being equal, to be coordinated in less centralized ways than less specialized systems. Under norms of rationality, treatment decisions are located at the lower levels of the organization, where the necessary specialized expertise lies (Hollingsworth and Hanneman, 1984).

On balance, however, the effects of the increased investment in human capital on levels of health in North America and Western Europe have been positive. Over time, this growth has been associated with an increase in the quality and efficacy of medical care. The expansion of biomedical knowledge has mediated the effects of general societal development on levels of health, for it is through the diffusion of this knowledge that considerable amounts of information about nutrition, child care, preventive medicine, and therapy have been transmitted to citizens (Novak, 1973; Smith, 1979; Woods and Woodward, 1984). It is also clear, however, that gains in population health have sometimes been constrained by the opposition of the medical profession to state intervention, which generally allows greater access to the benefits of medical knowledge and technology.

State Intervention and Levels of Health

The capacity of medical delivery systems to improve levels of health depends not only on the quantity and quality of resources in the system but also on the effectiveness with which these resources are brought to bear. As medical delivery systems become larger, more complex, and more specialized, the difficulties of matching resources with medical problems, allocating resources where they will yield the greatest return, and avoiding duplication and idleness increase.

In each of the four countries, the institutional arrangements for co-ordinating the delivery of medical services have changed greatly during the twentieth century. Group practice, health maintenance organizations, and state intervention are only a few of the institutional arrangements that have emerged. Of the various types of system coordination, again, we believe state financing and state control of prices and personnel to be most significant.

Governments in each of the four nations have frequently attempted to modify and coordinate the behavior of actors in medical delivery systems through the financial power of the state. They have offered and withdrawn subsidies designed to increase the quantity and quality of services, incentives intended to redistribute providers and medical facilities geographically, massive tax advantages meant to subsidize medical construction and medical consumption. Sometimes they have provided medical services directly to consumers.

The purpose of state intervention in the financing and management of medical services has generally been to improve the society's health by correcting "market failures" in the allocation of medical technology. We offer the following hypotheses with regard to the effects of these forms of state intervention:

4.8. net of other factors, the greater the state control over medical revenues and the higher the level of medical expenditures, the higher the level of population health;

4.9. net of other factors, the greater the state control of medical revenues and medical prices and personnel, the higher the level of population health; and

4.10. net of other factors, the greater the state control of medical prices and personnel, the greater the equality in the distribution of medical services and, consequently, the higher the level of health.

The control of medical revenue by the state does not, in itself, have any effect on the level of population health. What matters is the level of resources and the uses to which they are put. Thus, it is in the level of expenditures and in making medical services more egalitarian that the state affects health outcomes.

The increased levels of expenditure which accompany state intervention tend to improve levels of health by increasing the quantity and/or quality of medical services. These consequences follow because governments respond to political pressures for greater provision of medical care from populations that would not be equally able to realize their wishes through a privatized system. Simply put, state financing of medical care is frequently instituted in order to subsidize medical care for individuals who would otherwise be unable to afford it. Therefore, state expenditures for medical care often tend to supplement private expenditures for medical services. To the extent that they do so, state expenditures tend to increase the total cost of medical services and to widen the availability of care.

State financing eventually tends to give rise to state control over medical prices and the appointment of personnel, and indeed, in varying degrees the state in each of the four nations under discussion has been directly involved in providing certain types of medical services and in regulating the prices of others. State intervention tends to evolve in this way because control of financing is not nearly as effective in shaping system performance as control over prices and personnel.

Historically, European governments have long been involved in medical care, providing services especially to the poor and other "special" populations—veterans, the chronically mentally ill, the physically disabled, widows, orphans, etc. In Europe as well as the United States various types of medical insurance systems have been devised to share the risks of illness and injury across wide segments of the population and so increase access to care. In each case, the state has eventually used insurance systems or some form of third-party reimbursement to modify system behavior, either by direct state control over virtually all expenditures (as in Great Britain and to a lesser degree Sweden) or by quasi-public controls over some expenditures (as in France and the United States). The inefficiencies of managing system performance simply by controlling revenues have encouraged governments to increase their control over prices and personnel. One kind of market failure—namely, lack of access to medical care by certain social groups—leads to recognition of another market failure—namely, inefficient allocation of resources. Thus, the state intervenes to coordinate resources.

But why should state control of prices, personnel, and other administrative aspects of medical delivery systems improve levels of health as hypothesized? This effect follows as a consequence of the performance preferences of governments, which generally differ from those of the private sector (Hollingsworth, 1986; Hage and Hollingsworth, 1977). Specifically, the performance goals of governments tend to emphasize the provision of a minimum standard of care for the entire population; equalization of access to care across social classes, groups, and regional subpopulations; and allocation of resources where they will pay the greatest returns in population health. Political imperatives foster policies that emphasize equality of access to medical care. Such policies increase the share of medical care for low-income groups, which tend to have the greatest need for medical services and often benefit the most from them.

Social Development and Levels of Health

Clearly, then, changes in biomedical knowledge and the institutional structure of medical delivery systems do have consequences for levels of health, but these are not the only operative factors. Poor nutrition and housing, unsafe working conditions, environmental pollution, unhealthful life-style, crime, racial and ethnic discrimination, and war are only a few of the nonmedical factors that substantially influence levels of health (Woods and Woodward, 1984). So obvious and profound are the effects of these larger social forces on levels of health that the effects of medical knowledge and technology have sometimes been difficult to detect.

In the decades since 1890, both social development and modern medical knowledge and technology have advanced rapidly. In many ways these processes are so intertwined that it is inappropriate to ask whether changes in social development *or* biomedical knowledge and technology had the greater effect on levels of health. Social development was a necessary precondition to advances in biomedical knowledge and technology. Meantime, biomedical knowledge and technology have raised the standard of living and the overall level of social development. With regard to the effects of social development on levels of health—both direct and indirect—we hypothesize that

4.11. net of other factors, the higher the level of social development, the higher the level of health.

Recall that the term *social development* refers to a large number of complex changes centering on increased material standards of living, higher levels of education and communication leading to attitudinal "modernization," and demographic changes attendant upon greater longevity. Our hypothesis suggests that these changes tend, net of medical delivery system characteristics, to lead to better levels of health, mainly because rising material standards of living and levels of education reduce the risk of ill health by making better nutrition, housing, clothing, etc. possible. As we have suggested previously, many apparently independent effects of rising standards of living and increases in levels of education on health status are, in fact, intricately bound up with changes in biomedical knowledge. Rising levels of income and wealth are used to purchase not only better food but the preventive methods of improving health, which medical practitioners prescribe as a result of changes in medical knowledge.

The causes of health improvement in Western nations, thus, should not be viewed as purely a consequence of either social development or medical knowledge and technology. General social development improved levels of health directly and also indirectly, by contributing to the development of medical delivery systems. Medical knowledge and the delivery of medical services have also directly improved in population health and indirectly advanced the level of societal development. Instead of treating social development and medical knowledge and technology as competing alternatives—as some scholars have proposed—it is more appropriate to view these two factors as complementary. In the sections that follow, we will examine how societal development—particularly a rising standard of living—and the medical delivery system have influenced levels of health in Great Britain, France, Sweden, and the United States since the late nineteenth century.

Measurement of Levels of Health

It is extraordinarily difficult to obtain good data with which to measure levels of health through the past century. Ideally, one would like to have morbidity data, but such data do not exist for earlier periods. Even for the present era, good, systematic morbidity data are difficult to obtain for cross-national research. Therefore, scholars attempting to analyze changes in levels of health over time rely heavily on mortality data. Again, ideally one should focus on factors hypothesized to have had an impact in reducing the number of deaths resulting from specific diseases. Yet all demographers know that death often results from a complex set of conditions, not a single illness. Moreover, even in the present day, despite enormous improvements in diagnostic techniques, examinations of cause of death reported from autopsies reveal that the clinically diagnosed cause of death tends to be inaccurately reported in almost one-quarter of cases (Waldron and Vickerstaff, 1977; McKeown, 1978; McKinlay and McKinlay, 1977). Even so, mortality statistics do reveal important trends, and without them, it would be impossible to compare historical and international levels of health (Preston, 1976).

Developing an explanation for changes in mortality over long periods of time is like working with a huge and complex jigsaw puzzle in which there are missing pieces. One is always left with some uncertainty as to what the completed picture would look like. In research such as this, one must strive to be a good detective, exploring all kinds of direct and indirect evidence and pulling information from many different sources. One of the best indicators of changing levels of health, which we will add to mortality statistics, is height.

There is abundant evidence of the value of height for revealing the nutrition and health of populations during infancy, childhood, and adolescence. For much of the nineteenth century, many social analysts believed that height was the most compelling and revealing indicator of standard of living, and it has only been in the twentieth century that scholars have come to consider wages the primary index to the standard of living (Floud and Wachter, 1982; Fogel, 1986; Frisancho, 1978; Tanner, 1978, 1981; Keilmann et al., 1983). Fortunately, there is substantial data on the height of individuals across countries and over time, thus making it possible to assess the extent to which the nutrition and overall health of a country was improving, even when the mortality data are suspect.

Perspectives on Changes in Levels of Health

As we have suggested, Thomas McKeown, who has written extensively on the decline of mortality in England and Wales since 1700, has succeeded in convincing many scholars that biomedical knowledge and technology were of little importance in this reduction. In his view, mortality rates declined primarily because of improved nutrition. To test competing explanations, he entertained the idea that mortality declined as a result of reductions in the virulence of disease organisms, the development of immunity to certain diseases, and improvements in personal hygiene and public sanitation. After detailed examination, he concluded that none of these factors had much effect before 1935.

McKeown's methodology is to measure the decline in mortality between two dates and then to assess occurrences during that period which might have influenced the decline. In one study of the period between 1700 and 1971, he contended that 33 percent of the decline occurred prior to 1848–1854—in other words, before the development of most modern medical knowledge. But in most of his work he has attempted to measure the decline in English and Welsh mortality due to specific infectious diseases between 1850 and 1971. During this particular period, the standardized death rate declined from 13 per thousand to 0.7 per thousand, with 54 percent of the decline being attributed to airborne diseases, 28 percent to food- and waterborne diseases, and 18 percent to diseases from other causes. McKeown carefully dates the period when the decline of specific diseases occurred and determines whether the medical technology applicable to that disease came into existence before the decline. If a technology was introduced after the decline occurred, obviously, it could not have caused the decline. For example, he notes that the development of a public water supply could have had little effect in reducing mortality from airborne diseases, and as long as water supplies were polluted, personal hygiene could not protect against cholera and typhoid fever. According to McKeown, under these circumstances, "the washing of hands was about as effective as the wringing of hands" (McKeown, 1978:540), though in some of his work he acknowledges that specific sanitary reforms did help reduce deaths from cholera, typhus, and typhoid (McKeown and Record, 1962; McKeown, 1976; Woods and Woodward, 1984).

McKeown attributes much of the reduction in mortality in the late nineteenth and early twentieth centuries to the decline in respiratory tuberculosis (McKeown, 1976a, 1976b). Inasmuch as the tubercle bacillus was not identified until 1882 and an efficacious chemotherapy for tuberculosis was not developed until 1947, he concludes that the decline could not have occurred as a result of advances in medical technology. In regard to other infectious diseases, his reasoning is similar, and McKeown maintains that medical therapy and immunization had only a marginal effect before 1935.

Instead, McKeown attributes mortality declines to improvements in diet, arriving at this conclusion, first, by eliminating other explanations. Second, he notes the agricultural revolution during the eighteenth and nineteenth centuries, which accompanied the decline in mortality and increase in population. Third, he presents the research of present-day scientists who have concluded that malnutrition and infectious diseases are intricately linked and that reductions in malnutrition substantially reduce the incidence of infectious diseases (McKeown, 1976:136; Fogel, 1986).

McKeown's work is impressive, but his evidence and his methods are debatable (see Woodward, 1984; Woods and Woodward, 1984). For example, historical demographers are not at all in agreement about the causes of the dramatic population increase that began in the eighteenth century. Whereas McKeown believes that it occurred primarily as a result of a decline in mortality, H. J. Habakkuk (1971) attributes it to increased fertility (also see Wrigley and Schofield, 1981; Flinn, 1982). Unfortunately, mortality data are so poor in Britain before 1837 and in the United States before 1900 that historical demographers are hard put to determine either the level of mortality or whether it was actually declining (Fogel, 1986; Vinovskis, 1972; Easterlin, 1977; Lindert, 1983). For example, some scholars believe that mortality fell continuously throughout the latter part of the nineteenth century in the United States (Taeuber and Taeuber, 1958; Coale and Zelnick, 1963:7–9), while others insist that very little decline occurred before 1880 (Higgs, 1971:68, 1979; Meeker, 1972).

The best data for Britain before 1837 and for the United States before 1900 are derived from parish records. Some rather good parish studies indicate that mortality was increasing during much of the nineteenth century in the United States, even as food supplies had increased and prices declined (Yasuba, 1962; Meindl and Swedlund, 1977:398; Fogel, 1986:7). Indeed, several international studies suggest that the decline in food prices (and presumably an increase in food supplies) did not reduce mortality (Appleby, 1975; Schofield, 1983: 282; Fogel, 1986:9). On the contrary, a great deal of evidence suggests that the health of populations did not substantially improve during the eighteenth and nineteenth centuries, despite a better food supply. Obviously, the link between the increased availability of food and better health is more complex than McKeown's stimulating and provocative work demonstrates (also see Woods and Woodward, 1984; Oddy and Miller, 1976; Oddy, 1982; Beaver, 1973).

The economic historian Robert Fogel (1986) has used the scholarship of nutritionists to show that nutritional status depends not only on the amount of food consumed but also on the claims against that consumption. To determine the actual effect of nutrition on health, it is thus necessary to measure the net value of increased consumption after subtracting the claims against it. Physiologists and nutritionists have demonstrated that height and other anthropometric measures reliably indicate actual nutritional status (Eveleth and Tanner, 1976; Habicht et al., 1979; Winick and Brasel, 1980; Fogel, 1986), as long as the researcher also considers that height depends not only on nutrition but on age, existing disease and disease environment, climate, clothing, shelter, the type of food consumed, and the quality of public sanitation (Fogel, 1986; Eveleth and Tanner, 1976).

It is now clear that the standard of living—measured by increases in wages and available food—was rising during much of the nineteenth century in Western Europe and North America (David and Solar, 1977; Williamson, 1976, 1981a, 1981b, 1982; Williamson and Lindert, 1980; Shammas, 1983; Komlos, 1988). Nevertheless, in most countries height did not significantly increase, suggesting, contrary to McKeown's arguments, that the level of health was not very much affected—at least not in France, Great Britain, and the United States. For example, our best historical evidence indicates that the height of English working-class males hardly changed between 1840 and the end of the century, when there was a considerable spurt in the economy. Similarly, in France growth curves remained constant from about 1820 until the end of the nineteenth century, when height suddenly began to increase. And in the United States, the height of the working class actually declined during much of the nineteenth century but began to increase at the very end of the century (Sokoloff and Villaflor, 1982; Komlos, 1987; Floud and Wachter, 1982, 1983; Floud, 1983a, 1983b).

Obviously, increased wages and food consumption were not sufficient to overcome the effects of a host of adverse conditions. For example, cities grew at an unprecedented rate in the United States, bringing overcrowding that encouraged the spread of respiratory illness and enteric diseases. Widespread diarrhea and other gastrointestinal diseases diverted ingested nutrients from growth before and after birth, keeping nutritional status low and mortality high. Overwork of mothers undoubtedly retarded fetal development, especially when the insult occurred during the first trimester of pregnancy. No doubt intrauterine infections not only contributed to the large proportion of low-weight births and high infant mortality in Europe and the United States but "increased the incidence of birth anomalies that severely affected the respiratory, circulatory, renal, skeletal, immune, and neurological systems and thus undermined physical development throughout the first year, and often well into the second year and beyond" (Fogel, 1986:107). Moreover, the heavy intake of salt from meat and fish before the age of refrigeration probably contributed to gastrointestinal and cardiovascular diseases, and the consumption of lead, arsenic, snakeroot, and moldy food all had poisonous effects. Indeed, we have good reason to believe that the nutritional and other health insults delivered in utero and in early childhood probably affected disease levels throughout the life cycle (Ackernecht, 1945; Smillie, 1955; May, 1958; Kunitz, 1983; Fitzhardinge and Steven, 1972; Shapiro et al., 1980; Christianson et al., 1981; McCormick, 1985).

Clearly, neither a rising standard of living nor a simple increase in the supply of food was sufficient to bring about a decline in mortality. Biomedical advances, which began to accelerate in the late nineteenth century, had to intervene. Of course, the rate of decline varied from place to place and from one time period to another (Woods and Woodward, 1984)—as have disease patterns—and different forms of biomedical knowledge and technology have had different effects. McKeown is correct to say that therapeutic intervention, or "curative" medicine, had only modest effects on the mortality rate in the late nineteenth and early twentieth centuries. But McKeown has oversimplified the way in which nutrition influenced the decline in mortality. New biomedical information about dietary habits, public sanitation, immunization, and cleanliness unquestionably contributed substantially to the decline in mortality over the past century. In each time period medical science mediated between the rising standard of living and mortality in a pattern far more complex than McKeown has acknowledged.

The Decline in Mortality, 1880–1930

As we have suggested, McKeown attributed most of the change in mortality in England and Wales to the decline in tuberculosis, noting that improvements in water supply and changes in personal sanitation would have affected only food- and waterborne diseases and not such airborne diseases as tuberculosis. Elsewhere, however, the decline in mortality was related to other diseases, which were controlled because of advances in medical knowledge and practice. For example, Samuel H. Preston and Etienne Van de Walle (1978) report that tuberculosis rates were either stable or rising in France during the nineteenth century, while declining waterborne diseases—typhoid fever, diarrhea, and cholera—were bringing down mortality rates. The pattern was similar in Philadelphia and other cities in the United States, though smallpox vaccinations also had an important effect (Condran and Cheney, 1982; Condran and Crimmins-Gardner, 1978).

Although the exact mechanisms of infection by waterborne diseases were not known in the nineteenth century, the miasma theory of disease, which was widely accepted, contributed to improvements in water supply and innovations in the disposal of sewage. By the end of the nineteenth century, public health officials were very much aware that typhoid fever outbreaks and diarrheal diseases were linked to water supply. As city after city began to develop filtration systems and as physicians and public health officials preached the gospel of personal hygiene, mortality from typhoid fever, diarrheal diseases, and other ailments dropped dramatically. Moreover, whereas McKeown plays down the link between improvements in the water supply and the decline in tuberculosis, there is substantial evidence that the two were very much connected.

Food- and waterborne diseases such as diarrhea leave the host in a depleted and weakened condition, thus increasing the potential for respiratory infections. And indeed, the historical evidence demonstrates that as sanitation improved, deaths from tuberculosis declined along with those from intestinal ailments (Sedgwick and MacNutt, 1910; Preston and Van de Walle, 1978). These measures were preventive, not curative, but they clearly resulted from changes in biomedical knowledge that were rapidly diffusing throughout Western Europe and North America. The medical profession during the past century has generally been very much involved in educating the public about advances in biomedical knowledge. And it was the dissemination of new biomedical knowledge which did much to improve levels of health in each of the four countries during the late nineteenth and early twentieth centuries.[1]

This dissemination of new information was especially helpful for infants, young children, and mothers. In all four countries, local medical societies and public health officials began to publish pamphlets about infant feeding and to campaign against the adulteration and contamination of milk. Mothers were instructed to breast-feed their babies, to postpone weaning until after summer months, to use clean nursing bottles if children were not being breast-fed. Dried and canned milk, both less likely to carry the tubercle bacillus, became widespread, and pasteurization also became increasingly common, so that by 1920 the amount of milk with bacteriological contamination had declined substantially. Meanwhile, physicians on both sides of the Atlantic were active in education campaigns about proper diet, which reduced the incidence of scurvy, rickets, pellagra, and other deficiency diseases (Beaver, 1973; Winter, 1977; Condran and Cheney, 1982; House of Commons, 1904, 1910; Thompson, 1984; Woods, 1984; Smith, 1979; Dyhouse, 1978).

By the turn of the century, the link between the well-being of infants

1. Of course, the medical profession does not always embrace the lastest biomedical knowledge. On many occasions, epidemiologists have reached very accurate conclusions about the etiology and prevention of diseases, only to have clinicians object that laboratory scientists had not definitively demonstrated the specific pathophysiologic mechanisms involved! For example, in 1897 the New York City Board of Health made tuberculosis a notifiable disease, but various medical societies condemned the action and the New York Academy of Medicine officially opposed it. An editorial in the *Medical Record* called the action "dictatorial" (Winslow, 1929; Terris, 1980). In this instance practitioners were particularly concerned at the prospect of state interference between patient and physician—especially official state inspection, diagnosis, forced isolation, and mandatory treatment of patients. In other cases, the medical profession has resisted the epidemiological findings themselves.

and the health of pregnant women was clearly established, and many countries began prenatal programs. Early in the century the Local Government Board in Great Britain helped to set up prenatal clinics and home visitation programs for expectant mothers and families with young children. By the second decade of the twentieth century, the Board of Education established classes throughout the country to train mothers in the prevention and treatment of infant illness. These programs were fully developed in the 1920s (Smith, 1979; Beaver, 1973; Dyhouse, 1978).

In the United States, voluntary home-nursing programs spread throughout the country, and some local governments developed maternity and child-care programs (Schmidt, 1973). The United States Children's Bureau, established in 1912, became a key organization for promoting maternal health programs throughout the country. Eventually, Congress passed the Sheppard-Towner Act in 1921, which led to the creation of approximately three-thousand public prenatal clinics and sponsored over three million home visits by maternity nurses (Rinehart, 1987).

As in other aspects of the medical system, the kinds of programs adopted to improve the health of infants and mothers varied from country to country. The British employed centrally controlled and uniform but locally administered programs, whereas programs in the United States tended to be voluntary and organized at the state and local levels, with an occasional program supported by federal funds under the Sheppard-Towner program. As a result, there was more consensus about the British programs, and they tended to be better coordinated, but programs in the United States frequently encountered a great deal of elite bickering and were often frustrated by public officials (Rinehart, 1987; Lockhart, 1984). Irrespective of how the programs were structured, they helped give citizens access to advances in biomedical technology, and the net results were dramatic reductions in infant and maternal mortality rates. For example, in England and Wales, infant mortality declined 27 percent between 1910 and 1919, and in the United States, infant mortality fell at an annual rate of 2.5 percent between 1900 and 1930 (Fuchs, 1974:32; Winter, 1977:394; Haines, 1930; Smith, 1979; Baker, 1913; Meigs, 1917; Beaver, 1973).

We are not arguing that the "medical establishment" was the only instrument for the diffusion of biomedical knowledge. Schools, newspapers, churches, engineering societies, and many other types of voluntary organizations played an important role in disseminating information about how to improve levels of health. Our contention is that the greater the number of physicians and specialists, the more widely biomedical knowledge was disseminated.

Moreover, we are not arguing that the theoretical basis underlying biomedical knowledge had to be valid in order to improve levels of health as the knowledge diffused. For example, miasma and filth theories about the causes of disease were often more incorrect than valid, but these ideas led to practices that resulted in better water supplies and sanitation facilities and to drainage projects that decreased the number of places for insects to breed and feed—thus reducing the incidence of diseases carried by insects (Riley, 1986; Blake, 1956; Tarr and McMichael, 1977; Tarr, McCurley, and Yosie, 1980). Discoveries in bacteriology, physiology, and nutrition developed new information about diet, not all of which was accurate. But the diffusion of this information, not only by physicians but also by schools, food manufacturers, and magazines and newspapers, led to substantial improvements in diet and levels of health in the late nineteenth and early twentieth centuries (Apple, 1987).

Decline in Mortality, 1930–1960

Before 1930, the biomedical contribution to declines in mortality rates was confined very much to environmental control measures, immunization, changes in diet, and health education. Few diseases could be cured, and treatment was mainly supportive. Physicians could alleviate suffering, nourish the patient, and encourage the physiological efforts of the body to cure itself. Then during the 1930s sulfonamide was introduced, to be followed in the next two decades by other chemotherapeutic drugs and by antibiotics. For the first time, effective treatment of many infectious diseases became possible, and largely in response to these developments, between 1930 and 1960 mortality decreased sharply for every age-sex group. The decline was especially impressive among infants. For example, between 1935 and 1950, the infant mortality rate in the United States declined by 4.5 percent annually, nearly double the rate of the previous period. By 1950, almost 70 percent of all infant deaths in the four countries occurred during the first month of life from prematurity, congenital defects, or other causes relatively unaffected by advances in biomedical knowledge.

In 1900, acute infectious diseases, including tuberculosis, acute rheumatic fever, smallpox, typhoid fever, diphtheria, tetanus, polio, and pneumonia, were the dominant cause of mortality in all four countries. By 1960, improved nutrition, less-crowded living arrangements, water purification, public sanitation, immunization, and specific antibiotics had transformed the pattern of mortality, and chronic illness was responsible for more than 80 percent of all deaths. Mortality was now due to such diseases as arteriosclerosis (including coronary-artery disease), diabetes, arthritis, chronic obstructive pulmonary disease, and cirrhosis (Fries, 1980:132).

Decline in Mortality since 1960

By the middle of the 1960s, medical experts on both sides of the Atlantic came to believe that mortality rates were no longer likely to decline significantly. Infant mortality rates in the United States, for example, continued to drop but at a rate of less than 1 percent annually between 1955 and 1965. Many believed that infant mortality rates had reached the minimum level, below which they were unlikely to decline (Fingerhut, Wilson, and Feldman, 1980; Fuchs, 1974b:33).

Indeed, throughout the 1950s and 1960s, new medical knowledge had little effect on overall mortality, and in several industrialized countries, the death rate for males—except the very young and very old—was actually rising. Slowly, these findings began to shape social science scholarship about the efficaciousness of medical technology. For example, several studies, using cross-sectional statistical data for these decades, concluded that medical services were relatively unimportant in explaining variation in mortality rates among highly industrialized countries and places within these countries (Cochrane et al., 1978; Fuchs, 1974b). Some also concluded that biomedical technology had little influence on levels of health (Powles, 1973). A more appropriate interpretation is that for a very short period during the 1960s, medical technology had so effectively diffused throughout industrialized countries that international variations in biomedical technology and mortality rates were statistically insignificant.

Theory builds upon the description of observed phenomena, and so it is not surprising that during the 1970s a number of demographic theorists began to focus on the limitations of further decline in mortality. Specifically, some scholars maintained that biological senescence would prevent further increases in life expectancy. Each species has an inborn limit on length of life, for certain vital cells are internally programmed to reproduce for only a limited time, and the industrialized West, it was said, had reached that limit. The average life expectancy in the population would be unlikely to change unless major discoveries altered the basic biological process of aging (Hayflick, 1965, 1975; Fries, 1980; Keyfitz, 1978; Manton, 1982). Moreover, although advanced industrial societies had essentially reached the maximum potential for reductions in infectious diseases and maternal mortality as a result of improvements in hygiene, nutrition, sanitation, and antibi-

otics, societal factors (for example, smoking and environmental tox-
icological hazards) linked to chronic diseases were causing health levels
to deteriorate.

Yet despite the argument that mortality levels had reached a point
below which they were not likely to decline, the fact is that mortality
levels have continued to fall since 1965 in all four nations for various
age groups. For example, following a very slow annual decline in infant
mortality of only 0.6 percent annually in the United States for the decade between 1955 and 1964, the decline during the next decade was
an annually compounded rate of approximately 5 percent for both
white and black infants. The rate of decline was somewhat more modest in the other three countries (Fingerhut, Wilson, and Feldman,
1980:7).

The explanations for this decline are complex. Certainly, continued
improvements in public education about prenatal care contributed.
Moreover, in all four countries, unwanted births decreased because of
better methods of contraception and more liberal abortion laws. In the
United States, births to mothers who have already borne three children, which are riskier, declined by 50 percent between 1965 and 1975
(Fuchs, 1974b:33). Also in the United States, certain organizational
changes in the delivery of medical services undoubtedly had an effect.
Medicaid and maternal- and infant-care projects lowered the direct and
indirect costs of prenatal and obstetrical care, both of which promoted
favorable birth outcomes, thus lowering infant mortality rates (Grossman and Jacobowitz, 1981). Several studies of these and similar programs have contended that the more medical care pregnant mothers
receive, the lower the infant mortality rate (Shah and Abbey, 1971;
Kessner et al., 1973; Erhardt et al., 1970; Erhardt and Berlin, 1974;
Hadley, 1982).

A recent Urban Institute statistical study of a large number of specific age cohorts in the United States, using data from 1968 and 1970,
unequivocally concluded that medical care significantly contributes to
lower mortality rates. Holding constant the effects of several socio-
demographic, behavioral, and environmental factors, the study revealed that, except for middle-aged males, a 10 percent increase in per
capita medical care would produce a 1.5 percent decrease in mortality
rates. For middle-aged white males (forty-five to sixty-four years old),
this 10 percent increase had twice as much effect, whereas for middle-
aged black males it had only half the effect (Hadley, 1982:169).

One of the surprising trends in recent years has been the sharp reduction in age-specific mortality rates of older persons. For example,
whereas the life expectancy at age sixty-five for white females increased
approximately 0.5 percent per year after 1930, the rate of increase was

1.3 percent per year during most of the 1970s. Moreover, mortality rates for both males and females over age eighty-five decreased rapidly, suggesting that neither sex group had reached its biological limits. Between 1960 and 1978, the life expectancy of white females age eighty-five increased from 4.6 to 6.7 years, or 46 percent, and for nonwhite females from 5.4 to 9.9 years—an increase of 82 percent (Manton, 1982:195). These improvements are primarily due to a decrease in the risk of death from heart disease or cerebrovascular disorders. Significantly, death rates from most other causes at ages sixty-five to eighty-four were virtually the same in the United States in 1980 as in 1965. Age-adjusted death rates from cancer actually rose between 1965 and 1980 among the elderly, possibly because this cohort had been exposed to cigarette smoking and environmental hazards several decades earlier (Fuchs, 1986:chap. 16; *New York Times,* April 16, 1987:B10).

There is no consensus among analysts as to why death rates from heart disease and stroke have decreased. A vast literature attributes much of the decline to advances in biomedical technology, but some cite alterations in diet, smoking habits, exercise, and other aspects of personal behavior (Crimmins, 1986; Rosenwaike, 1980, 1985; Russell, 1981).

It is doubtful that all the reduction in mortality from circulatory disease is due to changes in life-style. Very likely, better diagnostic procedures, such as angiograms, ultrasound imaging, nuclear scanning, and position emission tomography, have helped to identify latent defects, for which many new treatments—balloon angioplasty, clot-dissolving streptokinase, bypass and vascular surgery, defibrillator implantation, the medical treatment of atherosclerosis, and calcium blockers—have emerged. There have also been advances in the management of life-threatening events—educational programs to teach the public about cardiopulmonary resuscitation, the establishment of intensive-care units, and a variety of surgical and medical treatments for the management of myocardial infarction (Manton, 1982:221–22; Cooper et al., 1978; Gillum et al., 1984; Goldman and Cook, 1984; Levy, 1981; Stamler, 1981, 1985; Elveback et al., 1981).

Whether the decline in mortality from coronary disease and stroke is due to changes in life-style or to improvements in diagnostic techniques and treatment, the overall explanation is nevertheless essentially biomedical. Medical personnel and institutions have spread information about diagnosis and treatment and warnings about life-style throughout advanced industrial societies. More widely accessible systems have been most effective in diffusing the latest biomedical knowledge and technology throughout their societies. And yet, the explanation for the sharp improvements in mortality rates for the elderly—especially as related to cardiovascular diseases—remains problematic. We believe that biomedical advances are largely responsible, but there is a competing set of hypotheses. For example, several recent studies have found a statistically significant relationship between the biomedical condition of individuals at early ages and mortality rates from arteriosclerotic diseases later in life (Forsdahl, 1977; Marmot et al., 1984; Waaler, 1984). Hence, biomedical knowledge that improved the health of infants sixty to eighty years ago may well be having an effect on mortality rates due to cardiovascular disease now. Certainly, biomedical advances have probably improved health throughout the life cycle of individuals since the turn of the century in France, Great Britain, Sweden, and the United States. Contemporary declines in mortality at advanced ages probably result from the combined effects of better health, beginning in infancy, and better diagnosis and treatment now.

Some Quantitative Results

To assess the validity of our perspective quantitatively, we must develop an indicator or an index that measures the level of societal health. The natural logarithm of an age-sex standardized mortality rate, despite its inability to measure some dimensions of societal health, permits us to do comparable analysis over a long time period in several countries. And even if these rates are not the perfect measure of health, they can illuminate some of the basic causes and trends in levels of health during the past century.

We have used two transformations of the crude mortality rate to create our indicator. The logarithmic transformation of the mortality rate reflects the hypothesis that there are "decreasing marginal returns" in the relationship between the independent variables (social development and the structure of medical delivery systems) and the dependent variable (age-sex standardized mortality rates). The log transformation gives equal weight to large decrements of mortality at high levels of mortality and to smaller decrements at lower levels. The assumption about the form of relationship reflects the theoretical supposition that at some point there are biological upper limits to the span of human life and increments close to this boundary are more difficult to achieve than increments at lower levels (Manton, 1982; Keyfitz, 1978; Hayflick, 1965, 1975, 1977; Fries, 1980). This transformation also, as a matter of empirical fact, fits the data better than linear formulations.

The second transformation of the crude mortality rate is age-sex standardized to compensate for great variation according to these variables. That is, the very young, the elderly, and males of any age have higher probabilities of death than others. Therefore, it is desirable to eliminate the effects of cross-national and cross-temporal variations in the age and sex structure of a society's population. We could achieve these effects by controlling statistically for age and sex or by direct standardization, which is more appropriate to the small number of observations in our data. We recalculated the mortality rate for each nation and time point, using the age and sex structure that existed in England and Wales in 1931. The resulting age-sex standardized mortality rates (without log transformation) for the four nations are presented in Table 4.1.

In all four nations mortality rates declined substantially between 1890 and 1970. Although there is a significant difference between the highest mortality rate (in France) and the lowest (in Sweden) in 1970, the largest portion of the total variation is over time. In recent decades the long-term trend toward lower mortality has generally slowed, reflecting the difficulty of accomplishing major improvements at the margin. This slowing, however, has not occurred to the same degree in all the nations. While the rate of decline has been quite modest in the United States in more recent years and even retrogressed in France between 1960 and 1970, improvements were more impressive in Sweden and England and Wales.

Table 4.2 reveals the magnitude of the effects of each variable on the log-standardized mortality rate through zero-order correlation coefficients between the logarithm of age-sex standardized mortality rates and the various independent variables—investment in human capital and state intervention—and through standardized partial regression coefficients, which measure direct effects of the independent variables on mortality. As suggested by our theoretical discussion, physician den-

Table 4.1. Age-Sex Standardized Mortality Rates per 10,000 Population, 1890–1970

Year	United States	England and Wales	France	Sweden
1890	203	205	223	158
1900	183	185	215	154
1910	162	159	189	137
1920	148	129	168	126
1930	130	125	155	109
1940	113	115	147	100
1950	91	98	119	79
1960	84	87	90	72
1970	82	79	94	63

Sources: See Appendix 1.

Note: Standardized to the population of England and Wales in 1931.

Table 4.2. Decomposition of Effects of Variables on Mortality

Medical Expenditures	
Direct effect	−.48
Net causal effects	−.48
State intervention: price and personnel control	
Direct effect	−.57
Via medical expenditures	+.28
Net causal effects	−.29
State intervention: revenue control	
Direct effect	+.12
Via medical expenditures	+.02
Via state price and personnel control	−.40
Net causal effects	−.26
Physicians per 100,000 population	
Direct effect	−.25
Via medical expenditures	−.17
Via state intervention	+.21
Net causal effects	−.21
Specialists as proportion of physicians	
Direct effect	−.19
Via medical expenditures	−.15
Via state intervention	−.05
Net causal effects	−.39
Social development	
Direct effect	−.03
Via medical expenditures alone	−.16
Via state intervention alone	−.19
Via state intervention and medical expenditures	+.05
Via medical system variables alone	−.33
Via medical system and state intervention	+.12
Via medical system and medical expenditures	−.17
Via medical system, state intervention, and medical expenditures	−.06
Net causal effects	−.77

Note: The effects reported for each independent variable are defined as follows: the "direct effect of X on Y" is equal to the standardized partial regression coefficient of Y on X, controlling for the other variables shown; the "effects of X on Y via Z" is defined as the sum of all indirect effects connecting X and Y which pass through Z as the last mediating variable in the chain (in some cases, there may be several such effects).

GLS zero-order regression coefficients with mortality (* is significant at .05, one-tail): medical expenditures −.70*; price and personnel control −.35*; revenue control −.49*; physicians per 100,000 population −.53*; specialists as proportion of physicians −.81*; social development −.62*.

sity, specialization, social development, and centralized state structures are negatively associated with mortality. Holding other variables constant, state price and personnel control, medical expenditures, physicians per population, and specialists as a proportion of physicians all have a direct effect in reducing mortality rates. When other variables are controlled, neither state revenue intervention nor social development has strong direct effects on mortality.

Despite the inconsequential direct effect, it is clear that social development is strongly related to mortality. Its effects, however, are completely entangled with the structure of medical delivery systems. At the same time, the structure of medical delivery systems does have effects on mortality which are independent of the level of social development.

Significantly, these results corroborate our hypotheses. They suggest that societal development and the structure of medical delivery systems interact, that system structure mediates the effects of societal development on health. Imposing a structural-equation model (or path model) on the associations among the variables allows us to explore these processes a little further. Figure 4.1 presents such a model, with parameters estimated from pooled cross-sectional and time-series data for the four countries, 1890 to 1970 (for a discussion of the strengths and weaknesses of this type of data analysis, see Appendix 3).

Not surprisingly, the level of medical expenditure per capita has a substantial negative effect on mortality, net of the influence of social development and delivery system variables. The net effects of the state intervention variables on mortality are also substantial and negative but somewhat more complex. State control over prices and personnel indirectly limits expenditure growth and consequently slows the rate of decline in mortality (+.28). The direct effect of state intervention to control prices and personnel (−.57), however, more than compensates for the indirect effect. State financing of medical care has only modest unique effects on mortality (+.12) and little effect through increased levels of expenditure (+.02). Because state control over revenue is a major factor in the development of state control over prices and personnel, however, state control over revenue does have overall substantial indirect effects on mortality.

The supply of physicians has somewhat paradoxical effects on mortality rates. The density of medical practitioners has a strong negative effect if we control for the social development index, medical specialization, state intervention variables, and the level of expenditure in the system (−.25). Yet many of the indirect effects of the supply of physicians cancel one another. Even so, the total net effect of physician supply in reducing mortality is of some importance (−.21). We believe that further research on the relationship between the availability of physicians and mortality rates is warranted. Certainly, the productivity of physicians increased enormously during this period. For example, in the late nineteenth century, before automobiles and telephones came into widespread use, physicians made house calls and were able to see very few patients per day. Now, not only does each physician see more patients per day, but citizens see physicians many more times a year than was the case in the early part of the twentieth century. Perhaps a more appropriate measure of the dissemination of medical knowledge and technology would be the number of times patients consult physicians during a year. Unfortunately, this kind of information is unavailable for the entire period covered by this study.

The processes that connect increasing levels of medical specialization

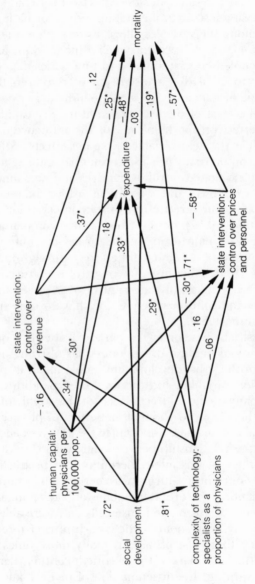

Note: The dependent variable is the logarithm of the age-sex standardized mortality rate. Standardized partial regression coefficients by the Parks GLS method are shown on paths.

*p < .05, one-tailed; N = 36.

Figure 4.1. Effects of Social Development and Delivery System Variables on Mortality

to declining mortality, as modeled in Figure 4.1, are quite complex. The model suggests that the direct effect of specialization (advances in medical technology) has been moderately negative ($-.19$). The effects seem to be relatively independent of both state intervention variables (the indirect effects combined are only $-.05$).

In view of the debate about the effects of the standard of living on levels of health, the social development variable is of particular interest. The strong historical connection between increasing levels of social development and declining mortality cannot be separated from the increasing density of practitioners and levels of medical expenditure, from the evolution of medical specialization and technology. Overall, the strong effects of social development on declining mortality in France, Great Britain, Sweden, and the United States have depended upon the development of the medical care delivery systems. It is perhaps possible that social development without concomitant changes in medical delivery systems would reduce mortality in other countries, but in these four countries the rising standard of living had little direct or independent effect. Instead, the effects of a rising standard of living were very much mediated by medical delivery systems to raise levels of health.

It is important to recognize that the medical delivery systems of these four countries have engaged in preventive, caring, and curing functions, which have varied in importance through the past century. For example, at the turn of the century, cures were relatively rare, but prevention was most effective. Once scholars recognize that biomedical knowledge and technology are not limited to medical intervention and cure of disease, perhaps we can better understand that changes in the standard of living, biomedical knowledge and technology, and state intervention have interacted to improve health and reduce mortality.

5

MEDICAL INNOVATION

This chapter asks how the structure of a delivery system influences the adoption and diffusion of medical innovations. Of course, many have studied diffusion processes (see Kalzuny, Veney, and Gentry, 1974; Freeman, 1986; Zaltman, Duncan, and Holbek, 1973; Katz, Hamilton, and Levin, 1963; Hamblin, Jacobsen, and Miller, 1973; Mansfield, 1968a), though relatively few have used a cross-national framework. Most have studied a single nation and emphasized the effects of societal values on diffusion rates. Several, for example, have differentiated cosmopolitan populations, which quickly accept innovation, from provincial populations, which are more resistant to change (Merton, 1957; Barnett, 1953; Becker, 1970; Mytinger, 1968). Our unit of analysis, however, is the medical delivery system of an entire nation-state, and we want to understand the effects of its structure. Hence this chapter attempts to explain cross-national variations in rates of adoption and diffusion of medical innovations through two characteristics of medical delivery systems: centralization under state auspices and investment in human capital.

There is no best set of innovations on which to focus. We have chosen three that permit both qualitative and quantitative analysis. First, we assess the impact of institutional arrangements on the rate of diffusion of smallpox vaccinations in Britain, France, Sweden, and the United States. Second, we focus on the speed with which various other immunizations diffused throughout these same four countries. Third, we consider the speed with which new drugs were adopted and diffused after 1962. Following in the tradition of Robert L. Hamblin, R. Brooke Jacobsen, and Jerry L. L. Miller (1973), we focus on the diffusion of each innovation throughout an entire society, as opposed to a single organization.

Human Capital and Innovation

In our introductory chapter, we suggested that high levels of professionalization and specialization tended to increase the innovativeness of a system, for professionals and specialists have higher levels of information and information passes rapidly among them (Zaltman, Duncan, and Holbek, 1973; Hage and Aiken, 1967; 1970; Katz, Hamilton, and Levin, 1963). Moreover, physicians are the gatekeepers of medical information for the society (Fuchs, 1986). Communication among physicians fosters greater awareness of innovations, both among physicians and in society at large, and hence greater demand for their use. We hypothesize, therefore, that

5.1. the greater the density of physicians in the population, the more communication about medical care and therefore the faster the adoption and diffusion of an innovation;

5.2. the more medical specialization, the more communication and therefore the faster the adoption and diffusion of innovations.

We should point out that each social science discipline has its own traditions for handling innovations, and there is no consensus about the definition of innovations.[1] We adopt the approach used mostly by economists, which identifies innovations with inventions or discoveries (see bibliography in Freeman, 1986). We also want to examine two approaches to diffusion, both the speed with which a society or an organization initially adopts an innovation (Aiken and Alford, 1970; Zaltman, Duncan, and Holbek, 1973; Shepard, 1967; Corwin, 1969) and the speed with which technology diffuses throughout the society after initial adoption.

High density of professionals and high levels of specialization, which

---

1. Examples of the economics literature are Smookler, 1966; Mansfield, 1961, 1968a and b; and Russell 1977. Some of the anthropological perspectives are discussed in Redfield et al., 1936; and Edmondson, 1961. For the political science literature, see Downs, 1976; Grey, 1973; and Walker, 1971.

often coincide and overlap, act jointly to increase innovation and speed both adoption and diffusion by fostering communication. As numbers of professionals increase, so do numbers of meetings, papers presented at professional conferences, and articles published in professional journals. All these forms of communication nurture innovativeness (Hage and Aiken, 1967; Crane, 1972). Specialists are even more drawn to such forms of information transmittal. Indeed, the relationship between specialization and professional activity is so close that one might think of this activity as an index of communication among professionals. Not only does communication lead to more innovativeness, but this kind of activity unquestionably generates new knowledge and spreads it around (Crane, 1972; Ben-David, 1971).

Marked changes in all these variables have occurred in the medical delivery systems of Western Europe and North America during the past century (Stevens 1966, 1971; Hollingsworth, 1986; Anderson 1972). The density of doctors relative to population has risen considerably, the proportion of physicians in a speciality has substantially increased since the end of World War II, and professional activities as well as the amount of money and energy invested in medical and drug research have also escalated. Again, however, the rate of increase has differed from country to country. In Europe, for example, a large proportion of physicians are not allowed to practice in a hospital and thus are denied a major avenue for integration into a communication network (Abel-Smith, 1964; Hollingsworth, 1986; Stevens 1966). In contrast, most physicians in the United States are affiliated with one or more hospitals and have more of an opportunity to keep abreast of current advances in the medical sciences (Hollingsworth and Hollingsworth, 1987). Other factors also play a part, however, among them the degree of state intervention, which could be identified as the compulsion factor, as opposed to the cooperation factor of professional communication.

State Intervention and Innovation

There is no consensus in the theoretical literature on the relation between state intervention and the diffusion of innovations. Even if we suggest that state intervention resembles centralization in complex organizations—about which there is much research—we find varied viewpoints. Some (see Burns and Stalker, 1961; Hage and Aiken, 1970) maintain that innovations are adopted more quickly in decentralized structures. In fact, considerable literature on complex organizations tends to support this hypothesis. Nevertheless, some scholars believe that centralization, although it may discourage innovation within an organization, might speed up the adoption and implementation of innovations from outside the system (Zaltman, Duncan, and Holbek, 1973; Wilson, 1966; Shepard, 1967; Corwin, 1969). Jerald Hage (1978) has reported that in some health and welfare organizations, centralization facilitated the adoption of others' innovations. Especially when the organization lagged behind others in level of technology, it tended to speed the introduction of innovations to "catch up." Centralized systems tend to wait longer to adopt innovations, but then, especially when the organizations lagged behind others in level of technology, they tend to implement changes more rapidly than decentralized systems. In a different context, Michael Aiken and Robert Alford (1970) demonstrated that American cities with decentralized political structures tended to adopt innovations more rapidly than cities with centralized political structures.

Most of the social science literature is concerned with the rate at which innovations occur or are adopted, rarely with the speed of diffusion throughout a society (Gray, 1973; Aiken and Alford, 1970). When we move our theoretical concerns from complex organizations to a societal level of analysis, however, this aspect becomes crucial, and we must understand both the speed of adoption and the speed of diffusion.

Thus, we hypothesize that

5.3. the greater the degree of centralization under state auspices, the less the interprofessional communication and the slower the decision to adopt a particular innovation; and

5.4. the greater the degree of centralization under state auspices, the faster the diffusion of the innovation once it is adopted.

Implicit in these hypotheses is the assumption that in a system dominated by a highly centralized state structure, the key actors are "plugged in," facilitating transmission of the message once the decision is made to adopt an innovation. In a more decentralized network, the message to adopt is likely to enter the network more quickly but takes a longer time to pass to all critical persons because it must go through a less-formal network of links that increase the volume of communication but decrease the speed of diffusion. In a market-oriented health delivery system, each individual practitioner, hospital, entrepreneur, etc. decides whether and when to adopt the new technology (Freymann, 1974; Ward, 1975; Alford, 1975; Law, 1974). In a highly centralized public system, however, the state is likely to mandate and to finance the technology in a single step (Lindsey, 1962; Stevens, 1966; Mechanic, 1972). Thus, the greater the degree of centralized state control over a medical system, the less the communication and the longer the time lag before adoption. In a hierarchical state system, knowledge of a particular innovation may be slow to arrive, or the system may delay introduction to evaluate the innovation, and the process of certification may take considerable time even if the levels of professionalization and specialization are high. Once an innovation is approved, however, the state system is likely to mandate and to finance its use, diffusing it in a single step (Lindsey, 1962; Stevens, 1966; Mechanic, 1972). Even in highly centralized systems, however, high levels of social development can pressure the state to shorten the lag time before innovations are adopted.

The Societal Context and Innovation

The number of professionals, the level of specialization, and the degree of state centralization are not the only factors that affect the rate of diffusion. It is also necessary to take the society's underlying social structure into account. The level of social development, the size of the society, and its level of social heterogeneity may directly affect the rate of diffusion. For example, a very large society with considerable social heterogeneity may, other factors being held constant, increase the probability of early adoption of an innovation, but these characteristics may impede intergroup communication and prevent value consensus and thus slow the diffusion of newly adopted innovations throughout the society. Increasing levels of social development—particularly higher levels of material wealth and education-communication—tend to encourage both adoption and diffusion. Higher levels of mass education and communication tend to reduce consumer resistance to innovative methods of treatment, and wealth provides the wherewithal to pay for them.

In summary, the relative rates at which medical innovations are adopted and become standard practice in national medical delivery systems are influenced by a number of factors. Within delivery systems, increasing levels of professional density and specialization tend to speed both adoption and diffusion, while higher levels of state centralization tend to slow adoption but speed diffusion. Social development, population size, and social heterogeneity influence the rates of diffusion indirectly, through their effects on the structure of delivery systems, and directly as well. Social development tends to speed diffusion, population size and social heterogeneity to slow it.

The Diffusion of Smallpox Vaccine

The smallpox vaccine provides an extended example of the processes at work in the adoption and diffusion of medical innovations. These processes—including making the decision to vaccinate, providing funds to cover the costs, and employing vaccinators—may each occur in the private or the public sector. Individual physicians may decide to vaccinate individual patients, or the state may mandate vaccination. Patients may be expected to pay for the vaccine themselves, or the state may pay. Each person may seek the services of a private practitioner, or the state may employ vaccinators. These alternatives can be coded on an index of state centralization, from the lowest level of involvement, in which all processes occur in the private sector, to the highest level, in which all occur through intervention of the central government. Between these extremes, the local or regional government may make certain decisions.

According to our hypothesis, the vaccine more rapidly diffuses throughout the society when all three processes are state controlled, that is, in Figure 5.1, when the processes occur in cells D1, D2, and D3. Diffusion will be slowest when the processes occur in cells A1, A2, and A3. In a small society with a high social development index, many physicians, and much medical specialization, diffusion may be rapid even if all processes do not occur in the D cells. But the larger the society and the lower the social development index and investment in human capital, the more necessary it is that the state become involved if diffusion is to be speedy.

The degree of such involvement, as we have noted, varies greatly among the four nations under study and within each nation over time. Large, ethnically and religiously heterogeneous societies are more likely to operate through the private sector (Weisbrod, 1977; Bendick, 1975; Hollingsworth, 1983; Hollingsworth and Hollingsworth, 1987) or through local or regional authorities. Historically, of course, the American system has operated in this fashion, whereas Sweden represents the other extreme, a small homogeneous society, apt to use central authority to spread innovations. Great Britain and France fall between these two.

Edward Jenner developed a technique for vaccinating individuals against smallpox in the 1790s, and his method spread to various European countries and the United States with hardly any time lag. Eradication of the disease, however, was slower, and variations followed the expected pattern. Sweden took the most vigorous measures against smallpox, completely eradicating the disease in the late nineteenth cen-

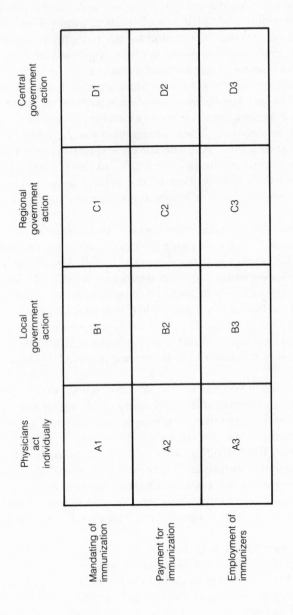

Figure 5.1. Privatization and State Hierarchies in the Diffusion of Immunizations

tury. The British had eliminated smallpox by the first decade of the twentieth century. The French and the Americans still faced the dread disease during the late 1920s.

After the first smallpox vaccination in Sweden, which took place in 1801, the practice spread very rapidly. By 1805, forty-eight thousand people had been vaccinated, and by 1814, 12 percent of the population. In 1816, the central government mandated vaccination for every child before the age of two, and by 1824, 88 percent of the children in Sweden were vaccinated. (Edwardes, 1903:45, 72; Guinchard, 1914:281; Great Britain, House of Commons, 1897:7993.698, 751–56). Both the Swedish state church and medical doctors compaigned among the citizenry, urging universal vaccination. The clergy frequently read from the pulpit a royal proclamation insisting on strict adherence to the vaccination ordinance, and pastors provided the public vaccinators with the names of newborn infants. In each vaccination district a physician, a midwife, or a parish clerk was appointed to administer the vaccine. So successful was the Swedish program that there were only two deaths from smallpox in 1846, compared to twelve thousand the year before vaccination began (Great Britain, House of Commons, 1897:7993.752–53).

Once smallpox was on the verge of eradication, however, enforcement of the laws became more lax. The epidemic that swept over much of Europe invaded Sweden in 1874 and caused several thousand deaths. Enforcement became strict again, and the government added a financial incentive, agreeing to pay a modest sum of money to the vaccinator for each person vaccinated. Hence, after 1873, the central government was deeply involved in the entire vaccination program. Even in the thinly settled northernmost part of the country, where roads were few and a substantial proportion of the Lapp population led a nomadic life, government vaccinators zealously carried out their responsibilities. In 1885 not a single case of smallpox was reported in Sweden. Despite a few cases in the next several years, smallpox had for all practical purposes been eradicated in Sweden before the end of the nineteenth century. It was a remarkable feat at a time when the disease was still rampant in much of the world. (Great Britain, House of Commons, 1897:7993.751–56; Guinchard, 1914:281).

The United States also followed the pattern predicted by our hypothesis, and as we would expect, this most market-oriented of the four systems was slowest to conquer smallpox. For example, in 1920 the United States had 110,672 cases of smallpox, the largest number ever officially reported there in a single year. There were more than one-half million cases reported during the 1920s, despite relatively high physician density, proportion of medical specialists, and level of social development. The low level of state intervention was responsible for the slowness with which smallpox vaccinations diffused throughout the society (*U.S Public Health Service Report*, 1940:2303–12).

No doubt the very size of the United States led to high reliance on market coordination. Whereas such small countries as Denmark, Sweden, and several German states had publicly mandated smallpox vaccinations by 1820, the United States had still not required them throughout the country more than a century later, even though the technique appeared in America as early as in most other Western countries. The first American was vaccinated in 1800 (Shattuck, 1948:180). Indeed, the federal government of the United States never issued a universal mandate. Except for select groups (for example, native Americans, military personnel, prisoners and patients in federal institutions, etc.), the federal government left regulation to the states.

Massachusetts, which during the nineteenth century was the most forward-looking state government in the area of public health, passed a law in 1855 which required children to be vaccinated before they were two years of age and prohibited children who had not been vaccinated from attending public schools (Hektoen and Jordan, 1909:50). But before the American Civil War, such compulsion was rare. The American states generally refused to mandate vaccination, preferring instead to require notification, quarantine, and isolation in "pesthouses" when smallpox occurred (Blake, 1948:1539). At the end of the nineteenth century, only a few states were mandating vaccinations for various populations. Even in states that required vaccinations, health officers repeatedly reported lax enforcement because of general apathy or lack of funds or both (Kerr, 1912:7).

In retrospect, the lack of uniformity is striking. By 1912 Kentucky had the most comprehensive law in the United States, requiring vaccination of all adults, all persons coming into the state, and all infants within one year of their birth. At about the same time, approximately one-third of the states provided free vaccinations for those who could prove they were indigent. A number of states required vaccination as a prerequisite for attending schools, but in the state of New York, even that provision applied only to cities of a certain size. Some states simply granted local school boards the option of requiring vaccinations for entry into schools, and many communities refused to exercise the option. And in stark contrast to the trends widespread in Europe, four states (Arizona, Minnesota, North Dakota, and Utah) had statutory provisions *against* compulsory vaccinations. It was largely because of this lack of government coordination that there were ten thousand cases of smallpox in the United States as late as 1939, the beginning of

World War II (Fowler, 1927:2; *U.S. Public Health Service Report*, 1940; Kerr, 1912).

Britain falls between the two poles of Sweden and the United States. While vaccinations were quickly diffusing through the Scandinavian countries and several German states, the British responded somewhat slowly, even though the technique had been developed in Britain and even though a commission of the Royal College of Physicians had strongly endorsed the idea of vaccinations in 1807 (Dixon, 1962:278; Simon, 1857; Great Britain, House of Commons, 1889:5845.71). For some years Parliament expressed very little interest in the issue.

It was the medical profession, acting through the Epidemiological Society, which finally persuaded Parliament to make vaccinations compulsory. The law enacted in 1853 required vaccination of all infants within three months of their birth. Parents who failed to comply were to be fined twenty shillings—a large sum at the time. Despite this penalty, however, the number of people vaccinated was not extensive until 1867 when Parliament provided for paid vaccination officers. At first, local boards of guardians were only *authorized* to appoint these officers, but in 1871 Parliament made the appointment compulsory throughout the country. Because they were paid a specified sum of money for each vaccination, public vaccinators had an incentive to implement the legislation. Soon it became common practice for vaccinators to seek out newborn infants in their homes, and within several years, almost 95 percent of infants were vaccinated (Forbes, 1937:175; Lambert, 1962).

As in Sweden, once the incidence of smallpox declined, enforcement became somewhat lax, and the proportion of infants who were vaccinated declined. Responding to fears of adverse reactions to the vaccine, moreover, Parliament in 1898 permitted parents to exempt their children from vaccinations for "reasons of conscience" (Forbes, 1937:175). Even so, the number of infants vaccinated remained very high, and morbidity and mortality statistics from smallpox continued to decline. Shortly after the turn of the twentieth century—when over 70,000 cases were still occurring annually in the United States—Britain had virtually eliminated smallpox (Dauer, 1940:2306; Great Britain, House of Commons, 1910:5312:xxx; Edwardes, 1903:73; Great Britain, Ministry of Health, 1931:6).

The French followed closer to the American path. By the end of the nineteenth century, France had neither mandated vaccinations for all infants nor employed public vaccinators, but the central government did require children to be vaccinated before they could enter schools. In theory, because school attendance was compulsory, all children of school age should have been vaccinated (Layet, 1886), but France lacked the vigilant system of public vaccinators developed in Britain and Sweden, and so, large numbers of children went unvaccinated. The pattern of vaccinations was also quite uneven. In urban areas, where communications were best developed and medical professionalization and specialization were highest, most children were vaccinated (Layet, 1886), in rural areas far fewer. Overall, the incidence of smallpox remained high. In the European epidemic of the early 1870s, France suffered more than most countries: there were 221,417 reported cases of smallpox in 1871, and 58,230 deaths (Great Britain, House of Commons, 1890:39.241). And in the first decade of the twentieth century, the incidence of smallpox was even higher in France than in United States. Shortly after the turn of the century, the French government enforced the mandate more vigilantly in the military and in schools, but the local governments still dragged their feet. By the end of World War I, the French, through more state coordination, were making more progress against smallpox than the Americans.

It is clear from the example of smallpox how state intervention can influence speed of diffusion. From Sweden to Great Britain to France to the United States, there is a progression in degree of state intervention which precisely matches the progression in the diffusion of the smallpox vaccine. Just how important state intervention is for effective diffusion is even clearer when we consider that its impact outweighs sharp differences in social development, professionalization, and specialization.

Other Immunizations: An Exploratory Quantitative Analysis

Many new medical technologies might serve to demonstrate the validity of our hypotheses. Unfortunately, however, it is difficult to obtain sufficient data on most. Of those for which data exist, immunizations are especially appropriate examples. Several studies suggest that cost, efficaciousness, and risk influence diffusion (Zaltman, Duncan, and Holbek, 1973; Fliegel and Kivlin, 1968). Since immunizations are highly efficacious, relatively inexpensive, and low in risk (Albritton, 1978), we are able to hold these variables constant. Other scholarship suggests that the values of elites affect diffusion (Barnett, 1953; Katz, Hamilton, and Levin, 1963; Hage and Dewar, 1973; Kaluzny, Veney, and Gentry, 1974; Rogers, 1962). Because the desire to eliminate death and disease from diphtheria, polio, whooping cough, and the like is virtually universal, the immunizations designed for this purpose have been little opposed, and this variable, too, can be held constant. Finally, the effects of many medical innovations are hard to track, but immunizations leave a clear trace in declining morbidity and death rates. A vast amount of cross-temporal and cross-national mortality data provide an excellent base for analyzing the impact of the structure of medical delivery systems on the diffusion of medical interventions.[2]

The data to be analyzed are neither time points nor societies but what might be called disease-country experiences. We are concerned with both the adoption and the diffusion of innovations and therefore with a continuous time period for each disease. These diffusion experiences can last only a few years, as in the case of the polio vaccine, which diffused rapidly in all countries, or they can last for many years, as in the case of diphtheria (Rosen, 1964; Parish, 1968). The duration also varies among countries. Thus our dependent variables relate to the amount of time required to complete the diffusion process.

Several methodological problems need to be considered. First, the data we use measures the effects of immunization only indirectly, through changes in mortality rates of specific diseases. We have chosen diseases for which we believe there are reliable mortality data in all four countries through the period. Nevertheless, the decline in mortality cannot always be attributed solely to the immunization (McKeown et al., 1975). For example, diphtheria mortality began to decline before the widespread use of an antitoxin (Rosen, 1958, 1964). Better sanitation, diet, housing, and other living conditions were probably responsible for some of the decline in mortality rates. Yet because we can time the intervention, that is, date the first use of immunization, it is possible to gauge the effects on mortality rates.

A second difficulty is determining the end of the diffusion process, which ultimately determines its length. The logic of an end point is the approach of some asymptote, but how does one define the correct asymptotic point? It is not the complete absence of deaths or disease cases. For most diseases, complete eradication may never be reached (Top and Wehrle, 1976; Hoeprich, 1976; Youmans, Patterson, and Sommers, 1975). For this reason, it seems more appropriate to speak of a steady state as a means of measuring the end of diffusion. The definition of a steady state for a particular disease is in part a function of the efficacy of the medical intervention and in part a function of the nature of the disease. For most diseases, we chose either five or ten deaths

2. The mortality and population data for this chapter were gathered from official statistics in each country and from the United Nations publication *The Demographic Yearbook*. For the United States, the most useful source was *The Historical Statistics of the United States* and the Census Bureau, *Mortality Statistics*. For Great Britain, the data, limited to England and Wales, were collected from the annual report of the Registrar General, *Statistical Review*. The French data were from the *Annuaire statistique de la France*, and the Swedish from *Historisk statistisk for sverige* and *Statistisk arsbok*.

per million population as a criterion for the end of the diffusion episode.

Once the duration of diffusion has been identified, a variety of statistical approaches to test the effects of social development, medical professionalization, and state intervention might apply. One common approach is to fit the time-series data on mortality rates for each nation-disease episode to a curve (most commonly the negative logistic) and then treat the estimated slopes of the logistics as the dependent variable (Hamblin et al. 1973; Griliches, 1957). We found this method unsatisfactory because the curves of mortality rates with respect to time are considerably less orderly than data on adoption of innovations in closed populations. Alternatively, event-history models can be applied to the analysis of the distribution of diffusion-event durations to estimate intervention effects (Tuma and Hannan, 1984). Such "survival" models are extremely powerful and flexible but too demanding of the accuracy and quantity of data available. Consequently, we adopted the simpler (and, we hope, more robust, if not precise) procedure of simple linear regression of the durations of episodes (measured in years) on the average scores of independent variables during the diffusion period.

Because it was possible to confound the effects of social development, specialization, and state intervention, it was important to select innovations that occurred at different times. We tried to select medical interventions that were spread throughout the period between 1890 and 1970, but because of the timing at which vaccines were developed, a high proportion of the interventions were concentrated in the 1920s (diphtheria and whooping cough) and the 1950s and 1960s (polio and measles).

Tuberculosis is an exception in our data set. The French developed a vaccine against tuberculosis during the 1920s, but it was not very efficacious and was hardly used outside France (Parish, 1968). Thus, we have not incorporated the tuberculosis vaccine into our analysis. During the 1940s, however, a new treatment emerged—a chemotherapy so effective that no one receiving the treatment, most authorities agree, should die from tuberculosis (Johnston and Wildrick, 1974). We have followed the diffusion of this treatment by observing the subsequent decline in tuberculosis mortality. As we collected our data, another difficulty occurred. Mortality data were occasionally difficult to obtain for the period prior to World War II. In general, each country monitored certain diseases more carefully than others, and they did not always share the same concerns (Brand, 1965; Rosenkrantz, 1972). As a consequence, it was not possible to include mortality due to tetanus for France (see Table 5.1).

Table 5.1. Immunization Adoption and Diffusion

Immunization	United States	Great Britain	France	Sweden
	Years to adoption			
Diphtheria	0	1	1	0
Tetanus	0	0	NA	1
Whooping cough	0	1	4	0
Tuberculosis treatment	0	0	0	0
Polio	0	0	6	0
Measles	4	5	0	0
	Years to diffusion			
Diphtheria	32 (1922–1954)	29 (1923–1952)	35 (1923–1958)	28 (1922–1950)
Tetanus	37 (1927–1964)	27 (1927–1954)	NA	27 (1928–1955)
Whooping cough	33 (1926–1959)	32 (1927–1959)	40 (1930–1970)	28 (1926–1954)
Tuberculosis treatment	19 (1947–1966)	19 (1947–1966)	26 (1947–1973)	20 (1947–1967)
Polio	11 (1953–1964)	11 (1953–1964)	12 (1959–1971)	9 (1953–1962)
Measles	4 (1964–1968)	7 (1965–1972)	10 (1960–1970)	4 (1960–1964)

Trends in Immunization

During the twentieth century, highly industrial countries have converged toward similar state intervention and investment in human capital, though some variation of course persists. The upward trend in social development, state intervention, and medical specialization in all these nations has reduced the time required for immunization to be implemented after adoption. By 1900 the technique for immunizing populations against diphtheria was already understood, but it was two decades before it could be sufficiently developed and refined. Widespread immunization against diphtheria did not begin until 1920 (Rosen, 1958, 1964), and several more decades passed before the disease was eliminated. By the 1950s, however, the level of knowledge and communication had increased so much that the polio vaccine quickly diffused in all four countries. As knowledge and communication continue to increase, we would expect technologies to diffuse even more rapidly, especially if they are highly efficacious, low in risk, inexpensive, and easy to administer.

As we study the effects of size, social development, professionalization and state intervention on the adoption and diffusion of immunization, it is necessary to keep certain caveats in mind. For example, diffusion may take several decades, but institutional arrangements do not remain constant during such a time span. Quite the contrary, they change every decade, and in some decades, they change a great deal. To compensate for this problem, we coded the institutional arrangements for each ten-year period, beginning with 1890, and then used the scores in two different ways. The time point immediately prior to the development of an innovation is used to describe the levels of state intervention and investment in human capital at the time of the innovation, enabling us to analyze the factors influencing the time lag before the innovation is first adopted by a country. To understand the factors influencing the speed of diffusion, we computed the average of each of our structural variables for the entire span of years needed to complete the process. Because of different rates of change, we measured dependent variables on a yearly basis and independent variables by decade. Our experience has demonstrated that institutional arrangements change slowly (Rokkan, 1970), whereas output variables such as mortality rates may fluctuate substantially in a short time (Keyfitz and Flieger, 1971; Preston, 1976). In determining beginning and end points for each case, we converted mortality data to five-year moving averages.

We must also consider whether diffusion actually occurred, whether immunization is responsible for the decline in mortality. If the decline is linear both before and after the adoption of an innovation, it may be impossible to determine whether the new technique had any effect. The slow but progressive decline in mortality might be due to improvement in the standard of living. Our data for some diseases shows a long decline in mortality before the introduction of immunization but a much faster decline afterward. Therefore, we conclude that there was indeed a diffusion process.

Finally, we must try to determine whether the relationships between the medical delivery systems and the dependent variables are spurious. That is, we need to ascertain whether variables exogenous to the medical delivery system more satisfactorily explain the rates at which innovations diffuse.

We observe from Table 5.1 that there is hardly any variance in the timing with which countries first introduced these innovations. Evidently, immunization does not confirm our hypotheses about how the institutional arrangements of medical delivery systems influence the speed with which new techniques are adopted. When they are highly efficacious, inexpensive, low in risk, demanded by most everyone, and easily administered, innovations are quickly adopted, especially in highly industrialized countries with excellent communication networks, high professional density, and high levels of specialization. We will test our hypotheses on adoption with a different set of characteristics later in the chapter.

The zero-order correlation coefficients between the speed of diffusion and our independent variables do sustain our predictions about the relationships among variables, however (see Table 5.2). The time required for diffusion is negatively correlated with physician density, with complexity (or medical specialization), with state funding, and with state control over prices and personnel. Furthermore, the higher the level of social development, the less time required to complete diffusion. On the other hand, the zero-order correlation coefficient between country size and speed of diffusion is almost negligible.

To press the analysis one step further, we have used a path model to estimate the unique (direct) and indirect effects of our independent variables on the dependent variables. The path model depicted in Figure 5.2 fits well with our theory. The decomposition effects for this model (see Table 5.3) reveal that the causal components of the total correlations are consistent with our earlier interpretation. The professional density directly and indirectly increases the speed of diffusion, though this effect is partially offset by an indirect effect through the two state centralization variables (+.24). Medical specialization also directly reduces diffusion time. Moreover, the total net effect of specialization on diffusion time is rather robust. Significantly, increasing funding by the state both directly and indirectly speeds up the diffusion process. Indeed, increasing state funding is the most important variable in accelerating the speed of diffusion. When other factors are controlled, the independent impact of centralized state control over prices and personnel is modest, albeit in the predicted direction of reducing the diffusion time.

Although these statistical analyses fit our hypotheses, the results should be observed with caution, for several reasons. As noted earlier, the inherent instability of the phenomenon and the necessity of using investigator judgment in fixing the onset and end dates reduce the re-

Table 5.2. Zero-Order Correlation Matrix for Diffusion Time and Medical System Variables

	1	2	3	4	5	6	7
Social development	—	.49*	.72*	.77*	−.01	.49*	−.77*
Size of country	—	—	.83*	.23	−.62*	.15	−.05
Physicians per 100,000 population	—	—	—	.43*	−.37*	.12	−.33
Specialists as a proportion of physicians	—	—	—	—	−.19	.42*	−.56*
State control over revenue	—	—	—	—	—	.07	−.42*
State control over prices and personnel	—	—	—	—	—	—	−.39*
Length of diffusion time	—	—	—	—	—	—	—

*p<.05, one-tailed; N=23

Table 5.3. Decomposition of Effects of Institutional Arrangements on Diffusion Time

State intervention: price and personnel control	
Direct effect	−.10
Net causal effects	−.10
State intervention: revenue control	
Direct effect	−.64
Via state price and personnel control	−.02
Net causal effects	−.66
Physicians per 100,000 population	
Direct effect	−.34
Via state intervention	+.24
Net causal effects	−.10
Specialists as proportion of physicians	
Direct effect	−.50
Via state intervention	−.02
Net causal effects	−.52

Note: The effects reported for each independent variable are defined as follows: the "direct effect of X on Y" is equal to the standardized partial regression coefficient of Y on X, controlling for the other variables shown; the "effects of X on Y via Z" is defined as the sum of all indirect effects connecting X and Y which pass through Z as the last mediating variable in the chain (in some cases, there may be several such effects).

liability of our data on duration of diffusion episodes. Because observations are few, relative to the number of effects to be estimated, small errors can bias, as well as attenuate, estimates of effects. We must, therefore, be aware of the possibility that the addition of a few more observations could change the results. Moreover, the disease-history episodes we have analyzed here are not "independent events" in the sense required by the statistical theory underlying the estimation of effects by the ordinary least squares regression method. That is, it is entirely possible that factors specific to given countries or particular periods of time, but not directly measured in our model, may be partially responsible for the results. Nevertheless, the statistical results are consistent with our hypotheses, though the instability of the results of our quantitative exercise can be appreciated when we turn our attention to the next set of figures and graphs.

In Figure 5.3 and Table 5.4, we explore the possibility that the effect of delivery systems on diffusions is dependent on changes in the larger social environment by assessing the effects of social development and size of country on the duration of diffusion. The effects of these variables, both direct and mediated by delivery system structure, are substantial, and in the predicted directions. The average size of the societies during the periods of diffusion has little independent effect on diffusion, but larger size is strongly associated with lower levels of state intervention and high levels of specialization, and through these variables, its tendency to increase diffusion time is substantial. General soci-

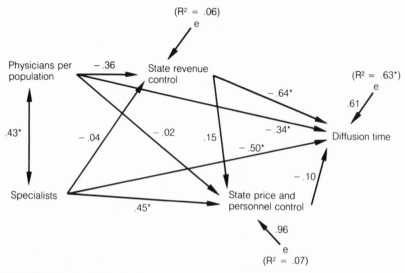

Note: Coefficients of determination are corrected for degrees of freedom. Standardized partial regression coefficients are shown on paths. Estimates are by OLS method.

*p < .10, one-tailed; N = 23.

Figure 5.2. Effects of Delivery System Variables on Diffusion Time

etal development (as measured by our social development index), by contrást, apparently exerts very strong independent influence toward reducing diffusion time, as well as creating indirect pressures in the same direction by encouraging medical professionalization and state intervention.

Whereas the effects of size and social development are as we had hypothesized, their addition to our statistical model seriously destabilizes the estimates of the effects of delivery system and state intervention variables. As can be seen from the path model in Figure 5.3 and the decomposition of effects in Table 5.4, adding statistical controls for size and social development has considerably weakened the effects of delivery system and state intervention variables reported in Figure 5.2 and Table 5.3. Indeed, although centralized state control of revenues substantially influences diffusion time in the hypothesized direction, the effects of specialization, physician density, and state control over prices and personnel are not consistent with our hypotheses. Moreover, the model in Figure 5.3 is considerably more complex than that in Figure 5.2, and hence the statistical estimation of the effects is more unstable. The two new variables are very strongly associated with the delivery system and state intervention variables and with national and temporal variations in the data. Given the small number of observa-

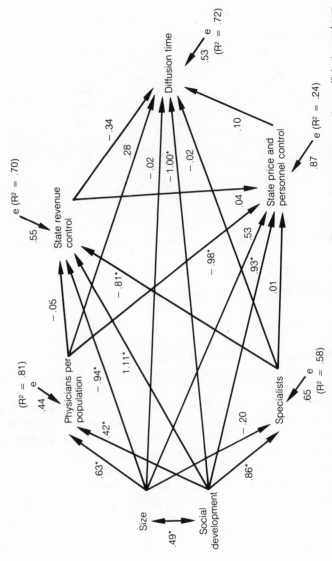

Note: Coefficients of determination are corrected for degrees of freedom. Standardized partial regression coefficients are shown on paths. All coefficients of determination are significantly different from zero at p < .10, one-tailed. Estimates are by OLS method.

*p < .10, one-tailed; N = 23.

Figure 5.3. Effects of Social Development, Size, and Delivery System Variables on Diffusion Time

Table 5.4. Decomposition of Effects of Social Development, Size, and Institutional Arrangements on Diffusion Time

State intervention: price and personnel control	
Direct effect	+.10
Net causal effects	+.10
State intervention: revenue control	
Direct effect	−.34
Via state price and personnel control	.00
Net causal effects	−.34
Physicians per 100,000 population	
Direct effect	+.28
Via state intervention	−.09
Net causal effects	+.19
Specialists as proportion of physicians	
Direct effect	−.02
Via state intervention	+.27
Net causal effects	+.25
Social development	
Direct effect	−1.00
Via state intervention alone	−.28
Via medical system variables alone	+.10
Via medical system and state intervention	+.21
Net causal effects	−.97
Size of country	
Direct effect	−.02
Via state intervention alone	+.36
Via medical system variables alone	+.18
Via medical system and state intervention	−.11
Net causal effects	+.41

Note: The effects reported for each independent variable are defined as follows: the "direct effect of X on Y" is equal to the standardized partial regression coefficient of Y on X, controlling for the other variables shown; the "effects of X on Y via Z" is defined as the sum of all indirect effects connecting X and Y which pass through Z as the last mediating variable in the chain (in some cases, there may be several such effects).

tions, the addition of these two variables to an analysis based on few observations destabilizes our estimates of the effects of delivery system and state intervention variables on diffusion.

Overall, this quantitative exercise suggests that the history of the diffusion of smallpox vaccine can be taken as characteristic of the diffusion of other inexpensive and highly efficacious medical technologies. The statistical results reported here are uncertain, but they generally support our earlier conclusions about the causes of variation in the time required for diffusion.

Pharmaceuticals and the Adoption of New Technologies

The qualitative discussion of the diffusion of the smallpox vaccine is consistent with out hypotheses, but the quantitative data on immunization lack sufficient variance for us to be highly confident about the impact of state intervention variables on diffusion. Perhaps another class of innovations and a different type of data can address our hypotheses. The pharmaceutical industry provides an interesting opportunity to assess the impact of state intervention on diffusion, even in essentially privatized systems. By studying the speed with which the British and the Americans adopted new drugs after 1962, we hope to show that diffusion is not the same for all technology. Moreover, the discussion about the diffusion of new drugs demonstrates that even in very privatized systems, there can nevertheless be a great deal of state intervention.

As a result of adverse public reaction to the medication Thalidomide, which was responsible for the birth of thousands of deformed babies, the United States Congress in 1962 amended the 1938 Food, Drug, and Cosmetic Act to give the Food and Drug Administration more control over the premarket testing of new drugs and to change the criteria for the marketing of new drugs. New FDA regulations imposed a delay of some years before new drugs could be approved as both safe and efficacious. Later regulations increased the testing period to slightly more than eight years (U.S. Congress, Office of Technology Assessment, 1981:34).

Thus, although the American medical delivery system is generally considered predominantly private, since 1962 the process for the approval of new drugs has been highly centralized and bureaucratized under the auspices of the state. The regulation of new drugs is as stringent as in any country in the world.

It is somewhat paradoxical that in Britain, where physicians practice what many Americans call socialized medicine and where almost all the hospitals have been nationalized since 1948, the introduction of new drugs for marketing was *less* regulated during the 1960s and physicians were freer to exercise their professional judgment in prescribing drugs than in America. Clearly, a system that is mainly private may have some aspects in which there is considerable state intervention and vice versa.

The ultimate power to approve a drug for public use in the United States resided with the full-time civil servants in the Food and Drug Administration whose careers depended on not approving a dangerus or ineffective drug and whose judgments were constantly scrutinized by congressional committees. In Britain, however, the approval of drugs during the 1960s was the responsibility of the Safety of Drugs Committee, a small group of unpaid, volunteer experts including physicians, pharmacists, and other scientists. The committee was charged with assuring the safety of drugs but not their efficacy. For a while, this procedure seems to have been quite acceptable in Britain, for many of the leading pharmacists, physicians, veterinarians, and pharmaceutical industrialists knew one another and were on friendly terms—not the case in the much larger United States. The more political and bureaucratic American system was biased toward caution and delay, whereas the British system, with less state control, moved more quickly (Wardell and Lasagna, 1975:98–99, 105–7; Grabowski, 1976:31–34; Dunlop, 1973:230–42).

Before 1962, the American rate of drug innovation exceeded that in Britain (U.S. Senate, 1973:9804; Wardell, 1973a). Indeed, shortly after the 1962 legislation, the Americans still had a slight lead. For example, between 1962 and 1965, twenty-four new drugs were introduced in both Britain and the United States. Two were introduced in both countries in the same year; the British were first to introduce ten of them, with an average lead of 1.2 years; and the Americans were first with twelve of them, with a lead time of 2.1 years. But between 1966 and 1971 there was a pronounced change. During this period, fifty-eight new drugs were introduced into both countries, fourteen in the same year, and in thirty-three cases the British introduced the drug first, with an average lead time of 2.7 years. There had been a distinct turnaround in the pattern for drugs introduced to both countries. (U.S. Senate, 1973:9840; Wardell, 1973a).

The change is even more marked if we consider all drugs introduced to either country. More than twice as many new drugs were introduced in Britain as in the United States bewteen 1966 and 1970. Of 123 new chemical entities introduced first in Britain, only 40 percent were available in the United States by 1971. At the same time, of 77 new chemical entities first introduced in the United States during the same period, 79 percent were available in Britain by 1971 (U.S. Senate, 1973:9427).

In some areas, the British lead was even greater. Between 1962 and 1971, in nine major therapeutic areas ninety-eight drugs were exclusively available in either Britain or the United States.[3] Of these drugs, seventy-seven were exclusively available in Britain for an average of 3.3 years, while in the United States twenty-one drugs were exclusively available for an average of 3.2 years each. In terms of drug-years of exclusive availability, the figures were 68 for the United States and 256 for Britain. Thus, in terms of both the number of drugs exclusively available and drug-years of exclusive availability, Britain approved drugs at a rate approximately four times that of the Americans (Wardell, 1973a; 1973b; 1975).

In the important area of hypertension, not one new chemical entity

3. The nine therapeutic categories were cardiovascular, diuretic, respiratory, antibacterial, antibiotic, central nervous system, anesthetic, analgesic, gastrointestinal.

was approved for the American market during the decade after 1963, while many antihypertensive drugs were being introduced into Britain (Wardell and Lasagna, 1975). One study demonstrated that in 1971 the British therapies of choice in several important disease areas were not even available to American physicians. Most American physicians were unaware of some of these drugs, but when they knew of them, the physicians wanted them for their own patients. Other areas in which British therapies were unavailable were angina, asthma, pyclonephritis, and gastric ulcer (Wardell, 1973a, 1975:166).

An FDA advisory committee was still debating the approval of the drug propranolol for the treatment of angina in patients prior to or instead of coronary surgery while the drug was so commonly used in Britain that failure to prescribe it would have been regarded there as suboptimal medical practice. It was finally approved in the United States, but only for minor uses. It was not approved for the treatment of angina for another five years.[4]

Some scholars, noting a worldwide decline in innovativeness even before 1962, which they attribute to the lack of advance in basic knowledge, maintain that much of the decline in innovativeness in the American system was not due to the more rigorous regulation of American drugs after 1962. Yet the interesting point about this worldwide decline is that the rate of innovativeness nevertheless varied from country to country, and this variation was related to the regulation of new drugs. The rate of decline was far more pronounced in the United States than in Britain and other countries where the regulatory process was less stringent. In those countries, such as Sweden and Canada, with essentially the same standards of safety and effectiveness as the United States, the timing of the introduction of new drugs was quite similar. (U.S. Senate, 1973:9386). Of course, economic considerations influenced the rate at which firms introduced new drugs into various countries, but the sheer size of the American market was extremely attractive to companies around the world. Because of the size of the American system alone, more companies would probably have mar-

4. The FDA was later to question the safety of some British drugs. William Wardell, an expert on the subject, has concluded that this argument is rather inappropriate: "In comparison with the size of the *total* burden of drug toxicity, that portion attributable to new drugs was found to be extremely small. . . . Britain experienced clearly discernible gains by introducing useful new drugs either earlier than the United States or exclusively. On balance, Britain appeared to have gained in comparison with the United States from its less restrictive policy toward the marketing of new drugs coupled with a more rigorous program of postmarketing surveillance" (Wardell, 1975:166–67). One may disagree with Wardell's assessment of the relative safety of the drugs introduced exclusively into Great Britain. Here, we simply point out that variation in the structure of the medical delivery system influenced variation in the speed with which innovations were adopted.

keted new drugs in the American system after 1962 had it not been for the restrictive policies of the FDA.

In 1971 Britain established a Committee on the Safety of Medicines, which replaced the voluntary system of regulating new drugs. The more centralized and stringent system quickly narrowed the difference between Britain and the United States in the speed with which new drugs were introduced (U.S. Senate, 1973:9381–481, 9802–61; Temin, 1980:148–51; Wardell and Lasagna, 1975; Wardell, 1975:165–81; Cuthbert, 1976; Graham-Smith, 1981; Whittet, 1970).

The differential in the time required for the introduction of new drugs in Britain and the United States sheds interesting light on our theoretical formulation. During the 1960s the United States had more physicians per 100,000 population, more specialists per hundred physicians, and a higher index of social development than Britain. Had these variables been decisive, the United States would have had a faster rate of adopting innovations than Great Britain. But the greater and more cautious state intervention in the procedure for approving new drugs was of more importance in shaping the time lag than the level of social development and investment in human capital. Despite the high level of medical specialization in the United States relative to Britain, several studies have demonstrated that American textbooks on pharmacology and therapeutics were substantially out of date during the 1960s and 1970s in comparison with those published in Britain. William Wardell, the leading authority on the subject, noted that "while all textbooks are out of date, American textbooks are so hopelessly out of date when used abroad as to be often irrelevant" (Wardell, 1975:165). In this area, communication was severely constrained by centralized drug regulation. Many experts have concluded that the cautious, centralized process tended to develop conservative therapeutic practices, with some adverse medical consequences for the American population (Wardell, 1975:165, 1973a and b; U.S. Senate, 1973:9802–13).

With several types of data and methodologies, we have focused on the effects of state intervention and other structural characteristics of medical delivery systems on the speed with which certain types of medical technologies are adopted and diffused. Vaccines are relatively inexpensive, highly efficacious, easy to administer, and (in the twentieth century) demanded by a high proportion of the population. In the nineteenth century, when the density of professionals and the level of specialization were relatively low and when communications were poorly developed, the smallpox vaccine diffused throughout the various countries at a relatively slow rate. And it was the structure of the state which did much to explain the speed with which the vaccine diffused throughout the system.

In both the nineteenth and twentieth centuries, immunizations of all types were initially adopted in all four countries soon after discovery, but the structure of the medical system influenced the speed with which the vaccines were diffused. Because there was greater variation in the structures of the four systems in the nineteenth than in the twentieth century, there was also greater variation in the speed with which the vaccines diffused.

New drugs, like immunizations, are relatively inexpensive, but unlike immunizations, they are demanded by only a small proportion of the population. Because they are less important to most people, relatively little information about them spreads through a society. Under such circumstances, variation in the structure of the state has considerable influence on the speed with which new drugs are introduced into a system.

This chapter has focused on relatively inexpensive new technologies. Other innovations may be both expensive and demanded by a very small proportion of the population. In Chapter 6 we demonstrate that decentralized and privatized systems dominated by providers tend to adopt expensive technologies much more widely than state hierarchical systems, which are more concerned with containing costs. In contrast to low-cost high-demand technologies, high-cost, low-demand technologies diffuse slowly in a state hierarchical system. Nevertheless, both chapters demonstrate that the role of the state, whether positive or negative, has important effects on the diffusion of medical technology.

6

SOCIAL EFFICIENCY

Talk of a "crisis" in the medical systems of industrialized societies usually centers on the rapidly rising cost of medical services. Less frequently discussed, but often implicit in the perception of crisis, is the slow rate of improvement in the health of populations in recent years. Taken together, these two aspects of medical performance raise deeply troubling issues: how much spending on medical care is enough? at what point are the returns on further investment in medical care virtually negligible in improving levels of health? how are decisions to be made about who will receive how much care?

The key policy questions facing Western nations go beyond the problems of the efficacy of medical services, on the one hand, and cost containment, on the other. System performance raises questions about the social efficiency of investments in medical treatment. For much of the twentieth century, policy was aimed at improving the quantity and quality of care, reducing scarcity. Now, policy must address the issue of how to allocate limited societal resources in view of the limited efficacy of medical technology.

In some respects, the medical delivery systems of industrial nations are victims of their own success. By contributing to the reductions in infant mortality and to decreases in deaths from contagious diseases, these systems have helped to increase not only the average age of the population but also the number of patients suffering from chronic diseases that are difficult and expensive to treat.

An elderly population is more than a medical problem. In all four nations, albeit in differing ways, the provision of medical services for the elderly has become a political issue and an important factor in increasing state intervention in the administration and funding of medical care. And as we shall show, state intervention has had major effects on system efficiency.

The efficiency of a delivery system is not directly reducible to medical outcomes and costs, even though efficiency is often thought of as a ratio between output and cost. As we have noted, the nature of the health issues confronting medical delivery systems has changed during the past century. In many respects, the "easy" problems, the medical knowledge and treatment that pay the largest returns in improving the general health of the population, have been solved. Those that remain are unlikely to be solved in the near future, and existing treatments are very expensive. For example, the causes of various forms of cancer are exceedingly difficult to discover, and treatments, even if effective, will pay smaller returns in terms of general population health than did efficacious treatments for bacterial infections. Moreover, even though it may be "inefficient" in societal terms to bring the entire force of modern medicine to bear on certain problems, in some societies there is pressure to do so. Heavy use of diagnostic technologies, vast expenditures on the maintenance of a few chronically ill persons, and massive efforts to prolong life may all be relatively *inefficient* uses of resources, in societal rather than individual terms. They may do little to improve levels of health of an entire society.

The development of medical systems in advanced capitalist societies tends to exert pressures against social efficiency in two ways. First, popular belief in the efficacy of modern medicine, together with the interests and predispositions of providers (particularly specialists), pressures the system to do everything possible to prolong the life of each patient. Maximum application of extremely expensive technology is brought to bear on individual cases. Second, the political strength of the medical establishment, coupled with consumer demand, undermines coordinative initiatives designed to achieve greater "social" efficiency.

The Concept of Social Efficiency

The efficiency of medical care has been a focus of a substantial amount of theorizing and research. Our approach differs somewhat, however. We have chosen to talk about the social efficiency of the system performance, rather than some similar-sounding but conceptually distinct measure, such as cost-benefit ratio or technical efficiency. Furthermore, we consider the entire medical delivery system in four countries, not the performance of individual providers, organizations, or programs. Many excellent studies of efficiency focus on the efficacy and costs of a particular drug, device, or treatment program. Some are concerned with the efficiency of particular programs (for example, whether outpatient surgery is more efficient than inpatient for a given procedure). Few, however, have studied the efficiency of national medical delivery systems, though discussions of the consequences of different payment schemes and other structures have some of this flavor.

The relative dearth of studies of the efficiency of national delivery systems is, of course, understandable. Neither the benefits nor the costs of systems at this level can be measured with great precision. Furthermore, the overall performance of an entire national–level delivery system is the result of very complex processes. The efficiency of the whole system is a consequence not only of the efficiency of each part of the system (each doctor, hospital, program, etc.) but also of the means whereby all the parts fit together.

Despite the difficulties of measurement and the complexity of the processes underlying the efficiency of national medical care systems, it is nevertheless important to talk about how systems have functioned in different societies over a long period. Such a perspective tends to blot out variations in the efficiency of individual providers, specific organizations, and programs and to zero in on those aspects that most influence total system efficiency. Thus, despite the difficulties, social efficiency must be examined at this level as well as at lower levels of aggregation. In other words, both types of studies are needed.

Another major difference in our approach is in the method of assessing the benefits and costs associated with delivery systems. Determining costs, of course, is relatively unproblematic. Whether one is examining the efficiency of a particular intervention, a particular program, or an entire delivery system, the resources used are generally quite obvious. All parts of the delivery systems absorb human and physical capital and raw materials, which can generally be reasonably summarized by a monetary amount.

The major conceptual difficulty, regardless of the level of analysis, is in determining the benefits, or returns on investment of resources in a given technology, program, or delivery system. For a specific medical intervention, it is possible to assess benefits by comparing the survival rates of a control group with those of the treated group. The "efficiency" of such an intervention would be the improvement in survival probability per unit cost, and alternative treatments could be compared in terms of their cost-benefit ratios. If units of improvement in survival probabilities can be assigned monetary values, then the return on investment in the intervention can be assigned a value.

Assessing the social efficiency of an entire delivery system is more difficult. First, there is no control group against which the performance of a particular institutional arrangement can be assessed. Rather, the performance of one system must be compared with that of others, and "adjustments" made for differences other than the ones under study. Second, the benefits, or output, of a medical care delivery system are numerous and diverse.

One might examine some direct measure of system output, such as the number of treatments delivered. This kind of data is relatively precise, but difficult to obtain in a multinational historical comparison. Moreover, this sort of statistic is too narrow to be very informative. What we want to know is how the amount of money spent on these treatments contributes to the level of societal health.

In a traditional cost-benefit study an economic value is assigned to the continuation of a life or the elimination of a death for one year. For example, we might assign the yearly income of a working person. But what do we do for individuals who do not have jobs or are retired? Or rather than use yearly income, pension, or other remunerative estimate, we might use the value of life, as is often done in court cases. Obviously, there are a large number of conceptual difficulties involved in any attempt to quantify the value of human life in this way.

In contrast, the concept of social efficiency presents fewer difficulties. We assume that each year of human life gained is a positive value—whether it is for a five-year-old, a fifty-year-old, or an eighty-five-year-old—and define social efficiency as follows:

$$\text{social efficiency} = \log \frac{1000 - \text{age-sex standardized mortality rate}}{\text{real medical expediture per capita}}$$

The numerator consists of the deviation of the observed age-sex standardized mortality rate from a baseline figure (1000 deaths per 100,000 population per year). As the age-sex standardized mortality rate becomes smaller, the efficiency of the system is said to increase, all else remaining constant. This part of the measure speaks to the level of societal health. The denominator is medical care expenditure per capita, in constant 1938 dollars. As costs increase, efficiency declines, all else remaining constant.

The social efficiency measure is an index of the level of societal health per unit of medical care system expenditure. There is, however, one last issue. The form of the measure we use in the statistical analysis involves the natural logarithm of the health-cost ratio. The logarithmic transformation is necessary because social efficiency is nonlinear. Larger changes in independent variables are necessary at high levels of those variables to have the same effects on social efficiency as smaller changes at lower levels. In other words, keeping a five-year-old person alive one year is much easier than keeping a fifty-year-old person alive one more year, and both are easier than keeping an eighty-five-year-old person alive another year. Age-sex categories are sensitive to these differences.

There are some difficulties with our measure. As we noted in the chapter on mortality, we do not have statistical indicators of the quality of life. Some people may be alive but almost comatose, and the quality of their life is dismal. To have a fully rounded measure of social efficiency, one would like to have data on the number of days of illness, but this information is not available over the entire time period in all countries.

The best analogue for social efficiency is the concept of productivity. In one sense we are measuring the productivity of the entire medical system, except that we are not taking the dollar value of the outputs and dividing it by the dollar value of the inputs. Productivity can decrease because medical costs increase faster than mortality decreases or because mortality increases with little change in the cost of care. In other words, our analysis of "social efficiency" addresses a somewhat different question from that usually asked by economists studying efficiency in the delivery of medical services. Our concern is with national reduction in mortality, rather than with the cost-effectiveness of specific treatments, programs, or organizations. At this level of analysis, social efficiency is the aggregate result of the performance of each part of the delivery system. We consider not the specific services provided but the health of the population as the benefit in the cost-benefit equation.

Renal Dialysis and CAT Scanners

We have chosen two examples to illustrate how centralized state intervention has enhanced social efficiency in Great Britain and how an emphasis on the private sector has reduced social efficiency in the United States. In these two countries the treatment of chronic renal failure with kidney dialysis and the diagnostic use of the CAT scanner are handled very differently. Kidney dialysis exemplifies how the goal of maximizing social efficiency at the macrolevel may lead to state rationing that limits the access of patients to expensive technologies. The proliferation of CAT scanners illustrates how the logic of market competition may result in the duplication of expensive equipment.

When the dialysis technology was perfected in the early 1960s, the British were pacesetters in the development of facilities for long-term dialysis. Early on, using funding from the central government, the National Health Service decided to provide the new technology to all who needed it. Before long, however, it became apparent that dialysis was extraordinarily expensive, and physicians in the National Health Service adopted a practice of limiting the technology to certain age groups—because of inadequate resources. In short order, a number of other countries had many more patients per million population using dialysis machines than did the British (Office of Health Economics, 1978). In most Western countries in the mid-1970s approximately 35 to 40 new patients per million (under age sixty and having no serious coexisting disease) were beginning dialysis each year, but in 1976 Britain had only 15.1 new patients per million population (Office of Health Economics, 1978:30). In the United States at the same time, there were approximately 60 new patients per million population (Office of Health Economics, 1980).

Of course, one of the major constraints on the number of new patients admitted to dialysis is money. Among eighteen European countries in 1975, the zero-order correlation coefficient between the number of new patients receiving kidney dialysis per million population and per capita income was .78. Countries such as Sweden, Denmark, Switzerland, and the United States, which had higher per capita incomes than Britain had many more patients per million using kidney dialysis machines. Britain in 1976 had 71 patients per million, Sweden 99, and France 111. But the United States led the world with approximately 170 per million.

Why was usage of dialysis so high in the United States? Predicting from per capita income, one would expect many fewer people to be using dialysis machines. The key is the privatized American system and its retrospective system of reimbursement, combined with the enormous power of physicians to shape public policy. American hospital administrators and renal specialists passionately advocated universal access to dialysis machines, and Congress responded accordingly, voting in 1972 to extend Medicare coverage for chronic renal failure to virtually the entire American population.

The British, by contrast, had a clear consensus for providing dialysis for otherwise healthy people under age forty-five but much disagreement on how to decide whether to provide dialysis treatment for older people (Office of Economics, 1978:52). The British state did not arbitrarily deny dialysis to people over age forty-five; the decision of which patients to treat remained in the hands of the doctor. The state did deny doctors the resources necessary to treat everyone in need of dialysis, however, and therefore, the medical profession tended to deny older people access to kidney dialysis.

As we have maintained in previous chapters, delivery systems with a high degree of state intervention tend to be quite concerned with both cost-effectiveness and efficaciousness of treatment. Hence, variation in the treatment of chronic renal failure has been influenced by variation in the costs of various methods. For example, home dialysis is less expensive than dialysis in the hospital, and the cost-conscious British have led the way with home dialysis. They have made extensive efforts to equip patients' homes with dialysis equipment and to train people to dialyze themselves (Office of Health Economics, 1978:36). By 1976 approximately two-thirds of the British dialysis patients were on home dialysis (by far the highest percentage in the world), whereas Europe as a whole had only one-fifth of its patients on home dialysis. An American trend toward home dialysis was sharply reversed by the 1972 congressional act. In that year approximately 40 percent of American dialysis patients were on home dialysis, but by 1979 less than 10 percent were (Office of Home Economics, 1978:38; Cameron, 1981:166).

Ironically, the British National Health Service, with its strong commitment to equality, has allowed less egalitarian access to dialysis machines than the market-oriented American system, which historically has had a relatively low commitment to equality of access to care. This particular technology suggests that the desire for cost-effectiveness may motivate state hierarchical delivery systems to constrain the diffusion of expensive technologies and to limit access to expensive treatment. At the same time, one could argue that restrictions to access on the basis of age do not violate the principle of equality but exemplify the necessity of rationing medical care, distributing treatment to patients whose prognosis is more favorable. Certainly this example illustrates a basic policy dilemma about state intervention, namely, nonprice rationing of medical care.

Despite the relatively low level of dialysis, the British have compared favorably with other nations in doing kidney transplants. Indeed, although the British tend to do substantially less surgery than the Americans for most types of illness (Bunker, 1970), they have performed more kidney transplants per one thousand persons than the Americans. Significantly, transplantation—when the proper donor kidney is available—is the preferred method of treatment. Because of the many complications connected with kidney dialysis, more and more physicians advise a transplant—when possible—instead of long-term reliance on dialysis. Moreover, a functioning transplant is considerably cheaper per year of of life than dialysis, and this is a major reason why the National Health Service has encouraged and funded transplants.

Thus, the search for less costly technologies can, in the long run, also lead to higher quality of health care as well, the real idea behind social efficiency. In market-oriented systems, however, lower cost is often not a goal. There is some evidence that because dialysis is far more lucrative than transplantation, for example, the American system was initially much less receptive to the idea of transplantation, even though the Americans generally do much more surgery than the British (Bunker, 1970; Office of Health Economics, 1980). In more recent years, Congress has amended the Medicare legislation to encourage transplantation. And in the United States today, victims of end-stage renal disease still have better access to treatment than in any other country (Held et al., 1988; Rettig and Marks, 1981; Rettig, 1986; Evans et al., 1981). Great Britain and eight other countries, however, presently have a larger proportion of their population with transplants than does the United States (Eggers, 1988).

The same sort of trade-off has occurred in the use of the computerized axial tomography scanner, another expensive technology. Even though the CAT scanner originated in Britain, it has been much more widely adopted in the more market-oriented and socially inefficient American system. The English company EMI developed the first CAT scanner and, for the first few years, installed all scanners that became operational (Banta, 1980). At a price of approximately $750,000 per unit, the CAT scanner was in the mid-1970s one of the most expensive medical machines ever manufactured. The annual cost to operate the machine in the mid-1970s was approximately $200,000. There was little room for such expenses in the typically tight hospital budgets of Britain, which had been state controlled since 1948, but the situation in the United States was quite different. In the market-based system of retrospective funding and competition among hospitals, the quest of hospital administrators for status and the demands of physicians have driven the acquisition of new technology. In general, the more expensive and highly specialized the equipment and personnel relative to other hospitals, the higher the hospital's status and the greater its ability to attract physicians, who admit patients. In this atmosphere whenever one American hospital acquired expensive new equipment, other hospitals hastened to catch up (Abt Associates, 1975; Davis, 1972; Lee, 1971; Jacobs, 1974:86). And physicians themselves have demanded that administrators keep up with technology, both because sophisticated equipment enhances their own status and because the proliferation of these tools increases their patients' access.

By the middle 1970s, it was not at all unusual for several hospitals in a metropolitan area to have CAT scanners. As late as 1978, there were only fifty-two CAT scanners in the United Kingdom, compared to over a thousand in use in the United States, over half of which had been produced in Great Britain. Per million population, the United States had more than five times as many CAT scanners as Britain. In fact, normed for population, the United States had more CAT scanners than any other country in the world, more than three times as many as any European country. Moreover, almost all this diffusion occurred before any cost-benefit studies of CAT scanners (Banta, 1980).

These two cases suggest that privatized systems tend to rely more on expensive technologies than statist-oriented systems. How much is enough high-cost technology if a system is to be socially efficient? Obviously, this is a very difficult question to answer. A high percentage of high-cost technologies are socially efficient in some settings but inappropriate in others. Certainly CAT scanners are extraordinarily effective tools for diagnosing many illnesses and injuries. And scans have been important substitutes for more complicated and invasive procedures. The British could undoubtedly make effective use of more body and head scanners. On the other hand, the Americans have had too many in some areas and too few in others, and scanners have frequently been overused (Kolata, 1981).

In Britain, where resources are rationed, most doctors believe that patients denied treatment for end-state renal disease are losing little additional life, that most of those who can benefit from dialysis or transplants receive treatment (Aaron and Schwartz, 1984). Yet, one American study has demonstrated survival for at least three years by 48 percent of those who received dialysis, 81 percent of those who received a transplant from a related donor, and 68 percent of those who received a transplant from an unrelated donor. All of these rates were for people over age fifty. Assuming that survival rates would be similar in Britain, one must conclude that some people over age fifty in Britain are permitted to die prematurely. On the other hand, many American physicians have been socialized to do everything of value to keep patients alive. And in Britain, Sweden, and France—where physicians are socialized somewhat differently—even if there were unlimited resources, it would still be considered inappropriate to treat many patients who receive dialysis or transplants in the United States (Krakauer et al., 1983).

In general, the British also provide less high-cost technology in other areas. For example, they tend to have too few intensive-care beds and to do too little coronary artery surgery. But there is persuasive literature suggesting that the Americans do too much heart surgery and have too many intensive-care beds. These and other high-cost technologies—unlike end-stage renal disease care—are unavailable to many low-income Americans, whereas in Britain access is based much less on income (Kolata, 1983; Aaron and Schwartz, 1984). Why do these differences exist? A great deal of the answer must be sought in the structural characteristics treated in this study.

Long-Term Trends in Social Efficiency

The level of population health in ratio to per capita medical expenditure, or what we have called social efficiency, declined in each of the four nations between 1890 and 1970 (see Figure 6.1). The Swedish case is perhaps the most striking of the four. The initial value of Sweden's social efficiency index is relatively high, primarily because of a remarkably low mortality rate. Among the factors responsible for this low rate were early and effective governmental public health efforts and governmental provision of hospitals and other medical services, together with the low population density and low rate of urbanization at the turn of the twentieth century. Over the long term, however, the social efficiency of the Swedish system has plummeted because relatively slow and linear improvement in societal health over the period has been accompanied by exponentially increasing medical costs. The same pattern underlies the long-term decline of social efficiency in all four countries, but Sweden exhibits the clearest pattern because of its initially low level of mortality and its prototypical pattern of exponentially increasing medical costs.

The American pattern was similar, although the social efficiency of the system was lower throughout the entire period and declined at a somewhat slower rate. Adjusted for age and sex, the level of health of the United States population has not been as high as that of Sweden, and the level of medical expenditure has historically been higher. As in Sweden, population health has improved at a slower rate than costs have risen, generating a steady downward drift in social efficiency. In both Sweden and the United States the decline accelerated slightly in the later decades of the period.

In the early decades the pattern was somewhat different in Britain and France. Both nations achieved continuous reduction in population mortality in these decades, with little or no increase in real medical expenditures per capita. In France, high levels of social efficiency reflected not high levels of health but limited growth in medical expenditures. As income levels rose and social insurance and other programs were introduced in the decades after World War I, the social efficiency of the French system tended to converge with that of the other nations.

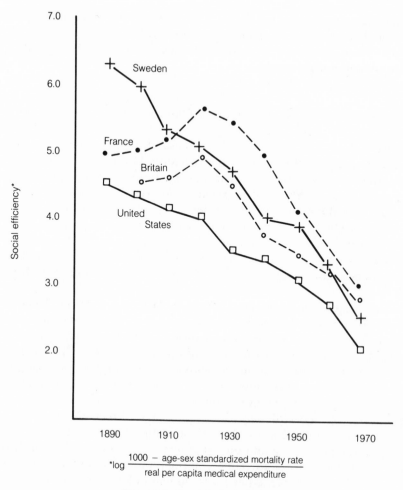

Figure 6.1. Trends in Social Efficiency

The British case, though similar in broad outline, is better characterized by three periods rather than two. Until World War I, real medical expenditures in Britain grew very slowly, generating serious postwar problems in both access and financing. Between the wars, the social efficiency of the British system converged with the others as expenditures rose more rapidly relative to the continuous slow decline in mortality. After World War II, the British system revealed the same symptoms as those of the other three nations, but social efficiency declined at a much slower rate than it did in the other three cases. Whether this pattern was attributable to the relatively poor economic performance of

Britain and consequent fiscal difficulties in the National Health Service or whether it indicates greater allocational efficiency under the National Health Service is an important question for our thesis, and we shall return to it presently.

Social and Political Structure and Social Efficiency

Figure 6.1 adequately describes the general differences among the delivery systems and their overall performance, but it cannot distinguish the effects of social development and institutional arrangements. We can gain some insight into the relative importance of these factors by reestimating the models of system development and performance used in the preceding chapters, this time focusing on the level of social efficiency as the dependent variable. The path diagram for this model is shown as Figure 6.2, and a decomposition of the relationships among the independent variables with social efficiency is presented in Table 6.1.

As this figure and table make clear, the largest part of the declining social efficiency of medical delivery systems is attributable to large-scale, long-term trends in societal development, the total effects of which are substantial. By our calculations, almost half ($-.34$) of these effects are independent of investments in human capital and changing patterns of state coordinations in the delivery systems. The other effects of social development ($-.38$) reflect its influence via the institutional arrangements of delivery systems. The direct effects resulted from many factors, of which the two most important were probably the aging of the population and the rapid increases in societal wealth. It is, we have noted, harder to reduce mortality in older populations, and wealth makes it possible to pay for treatment of long-term degenerative illnesses and chronic problems, which have a low social return. Social development, as a reflection of societal resources, also worked indirectly, encouraging expansion in the number of physicians and in medical complexity, which reduced social efficiency. Increases in social development led to more provision of medical revenues by the state, escalating costs and reducing social efficiency. State intervention in funding did lead to state control of prices and personnel, which tended to enhance social efficiency. When all the effects are taken together, however, social development accounts for a good portion of the cross-national and cross-temporal variation in social efficiency. The total net effects of social development on social efficiency were substantial and negative. Nevertheless, when the differences in the levels and trends of

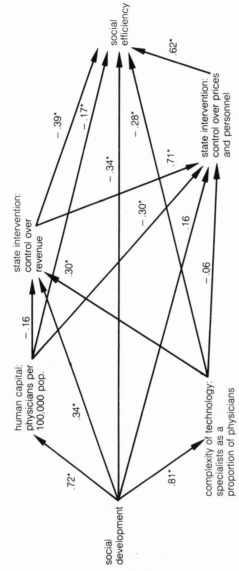

Note: Standardized partial regression coefficients by the Parks GLS method are shown on paths.

social efficiency = log $\dfrac{1000 - \text{age-sex standardized mortality rate}}{\text{real medical expenditures per capita}}$

*p < .05, one-tailed; N = 36.

Figure 6.2. Effects of Social Development and Delivery System Variables on Social Efficiency

Table 6.1. Decomposition of Effects on Social Development, and Institutional Arrangements on Social Efficiency

State intervention: price and personnel control	
Direct effect	+.62
Net causal effects	+.62
State intervention: revenue control	
Direct effect	−.39
Via state price and personnel control	+.44
Net causal effects	+.05
Physicians per 100,000 population	
Direct effect	−.17
Via state intervention	−.20
Net causal effects	−.37
Specialists as proportion of physicians	
Direct effect	−.28
Via state intervention	−.03
Net causal effects	−.31
Social development	
Direct effect	−.34
Via state intervention alone	+.12
Via medical system variables alone	−.36
Via medical system and state intervention	−.14
Net causal effects	−.72

Note: The effects reported for each independent variable are defined as follows: the "direct effect of X on Y" is equal to the standardized partial regression coefficient of Y on X, controlling for the other variables shown; the "effects of X on Y via Z" is defined as the sum of all indirect effects connecting X and Y which pass through Z as the last mediating variable in the chain (in some cases, there may be several such effects).

GLS zero-order regression coefficients with social efficiency (* is significant at .05, one-tail): price and personnel control +.12; revenue control −.42*; physicians per population −.78*; specialists as proportion of physicians −.72*; social development −.78*.

social development are taken into account, the structure of delivery systems also has considerable influence.

From the path model in Figure 6.2 and the decomposition of effects in Table 6.1, it is apparent that the two forms of state intervention have markedly different consequences for social efficiency. Net of other factors, state control over medical revenues has a moderately strong direct negative effect on social efficiency. Such fiscal involvement by the state, however, has in the long run been associated with increased state control over prices and personnel, which largely offsets the negative consequences. Thus, the overall net effect of state collection of revenues is very modest.

State control over prices and personnel markedly favors system efficiency, when other factors are held constant. Although this effect has by no means been sufficient to reverse the long-run historical downward trend in the social efficiency of medical care systems, it does confirm our hypotheses about the effects of state hierarchical coordination on social efficiency.

Increasing provider density (physicians per 100,000 population) has a moderately strong effect both directly and by its tendency to limit all types of state coordination. These findings support our contention that growth in the size and political strength of the medical establishment tends to increase medical expenditures more than it lowers mortality. In these four cases, the negative effects of the size of the medical establishment on social efficiency result from "excess demand" generated for "medicalization" and from resistance to hierarchical coordination of medical services.

In more geographically or historically limited studies, increasing cost and complexity of medical technology are often seen as enhancing efficiency. Our results suggest, instead, that the effects of specialization and technological innovation had an effect on the long-term cross-national variation in social efficiency, once the effects of other major factors were taken into account. The negligible net effects of the proportion of specialists on the efficiency of the medical care delivery system resulted from a negative direct impact, while specialists when mediated through the state intervention variables, had virtually no impact on social efficiency.

In two previous chapters, we described how state coordination shaped system costs and the levels of population health. The statistical results suggested that state coordination influences social efficiency by affecting both the costs of the system and levels of health of the population. Somewhat counter to conventional wisdom, we concluded that strong state coordination did not, on balance, increase costs. Rather, increasing state intervention tended to redirect expenditures, subsidizing use of medical services but restricting prices and the costs of personnel.

Strong state coordination increases the likelihood that there will be enough personnel, equipment, and the like in the right places. They are not unnecessarily duplicated in some areas or missing altogether in others. This sort of rational resource allocation enhances social efficiency by reducing costs. To the extent that such allocation is a primary consequence of state involvement in costs, it tends to encourage a wider and more equal distribution of access to medical care, with positive implications for social efficiency.

To the extent that limited medical resources are spread among a large number of people, however, rationing tends to occur. Immediately life-threatening conditions are likely to be dealt with before less-serious problems, and the less costly of alternative treatment modes for particular conditions are likely to be selected. Certain forms of expensive treatment for small populations are likely to be discouraged, and there may be waiting lists for some standard treatments.

Since ill health (and hence marginal return on treatment) is negatively associated with income, privatized systems tend, other things being equal, to provide excess care for the "well-off" and "too little" care for the poor. Where access to medical treatment is uncoupled from ability to pay (as in a system of equal, if limited access) treatments are more likely to reach those for whom they will return the greatest benefit. To the extent that state control of revenues, prices, and personnel tends to equalize access and to reduce the association between income and access, there is a tendency to allocate treatment in a more socially efficient way, as we shall explore in the next chapter.

The capacity of state-coordinated systems to implement changes more completely and rapidly than systems integrated by market principles also has some bearing on the relative social efficiency of medical systems. In some cases, particularly low-cost diagnostic and preventive procedures, the capacity of state hierarchies to compel compliance may produce substantial gains in population health over systems in which compliance depends on market incentives. Environmental medicine and the prevention of infectious disease are two very important cases. State hierarchical coordination can also increase social efficiency by retarding the diffusion of high-cost technologies. CAT scanners and other high-cost technologies are apt to be more efficiently utilized than they are in systems that are basically in the private sector.

In this chapter we looked beyond the quantity, quality, and cost of care provided to examine the comparative social efficiency of medical systems. The questions addressed are important both for general theory and for their policy implications. Policies that limit the growth in medical expenditures do not necessarily maximize social efficiency. Systems may spend too little as well as too much on medical care. Moreover, improvements in the health of the general population do not necessarily maximize the social efficiency of medical delivery systems. The same level of spending may have quite different returns in improving levels of health, depending on which services are supplied.

The root cause of the overall decline in the social efficiency of medical systems is not an "oversupply" of medical services compared to the marginal returns in the health of the population. Rather, it is the association of a large medical establishment with weak state intervention that has reduced system efficiency. Our findings suggest that medical technology and the growth of medical specialization per se have less influence on system efficiency than does the method by which these are coordinated—by the private sector or by the state.

7

EQUAL CARE AND
UNEQUAL HEALTH

In virtually all Western societies, the per capita consumption of medical care has increased markedly in this century. People visit physicians more frequently and receive more extensive and intensive treatment than previously. The increasing quantity and quality of medical care delivered, however, has not eliminated inequality in the distribution of health among the members of these societies. Within countries, various racial, ethnic, and regional groups have long been in substantially poorer health than others, and in most countries good health and long life remain associated with higher social class.

In this chapter we will explore some of the connections between the institutional arrangements of medical delivery systems and variations in the distribution of medical services among regions on social classes and in levels of health among social classes or income groups. Only in the United States and Great Britain do we have sufficient statistical data for long periods, and we will therefore limit our discussion to these two countries, although our theoretical propositions unquestionably have wider applicability.

For some years, the literature in the social sciences has emphasized the importance of differentiating among types of equality. For example, we might consider the right of equal access to some good. As economists recognize, markets sometimes fail. In such cases neoclassical economists consider state intervention to be justified in order to provide access for certain groups who would otherwise be without medical services. Traditionally, the state has provided treatment for certain types of chronic and catastrophic illnesses—especially for the indigent. In the United States, the rationale for Medicare and Medicaid was the lack of access to medical services by the elderly and the poor. Nevertheless, the question remains whether state intervention leads to greater equality of access. Another aspect of equality is equal spatial distribution of resources, which exists when the same resources are distributed to all individuals and groups. Equality in utilization of resources assumes not only that people have equal access to some· good that is equally distributed to all but also that people utilize the service equally. Finally, equality of results confronts the question of whether people have the same levels of health even when there is equal access to some good, equal distribution of resources, and equal utilization rates. In the past, many scholars have assumed that equality of access and equality in the distribution of resources would produce equality of results. As we shall see, we probably need to rethink this assumption insofar as health and other social services are concerned (Coleman et al., 1966; Coleman, 1968, 1973; Jencks et al. 1972; Bowles and Gintis, 1976).

State Intervention, Medical Complexity, and Equality of Health

In Chapter 1, we hypothesized that the more highly specialized a medical delivery system and the lower the degree of state intervention, all other things being equal, the less egalitarian would be their outcomes. The connections between equal levels of health among social classes or income groups and the characteristics of medical delivery systems are quite involved. In particular, the connections between state intervention and equality in the *access* to medical care are expected to be far stronger than the connections between state intervention and equality in *levels of health*. This crucial distinction is perhaps best seen in an exploration of how state intervention influences equality.

The role of human capital becomes more complicated as medical care becomes more complex. It is relatively easy to have general practitioners in all parts of the country but much more difficult to have highly specialized and intensive services everywhere. Holding other factors constant, high levels of medical specialization tend to have non-neutral distributional consequences. In a market-oriented system, the increased unit cost of specialized medicine may be expected to widen the gap in utilization rates between income groups (because of ability to pay) and social classes (because of different levels of understanding, trust, and sophistication). These differences in the propensity to utilize costly medical services may be expected over time to generate inequalities in access to and distribution of medical resources across social strata and geographical space.

Specialized medical treatment consists of a large number of independent, complex, and differentiated technologies, which tend to become concentrated in large organizations. In market-oriented systems, such concentrations tend to be located in or near high-income areas as well. This pattern increases the "transaction costs" of low-income consumers who live far from these centers, reducing their access to treatment. Low-income people are less able to find the right specialist and even less able to find the best specialist in the field. Typically, upper-income groups not only live closer to centers of specialization but are better able to evaluate physicians and hospitals because they have higher levels of education. And of course, upper-income groups can more easily afford to pay for high-quality care.

Although in market-oriented systems increased medical specialization and more complex and costly technologies may be expected to create greater regional and social inequalities of access, resource distribution, and utilization, the consequences for health outcomes are less obvious. High levels of specialization and concentration foster the development of complex diagnostic technologies, which are widely believed to be highly efficacious. Because these technologies are also capital and knowledge intensive and tailored to the medical needs of high-income consumers, their impact in narrowing social class and geographical inequalities in levels of health are somewhat suspect. In other words, specialization may tend to increase the cost and complexity of medical care and to increase distributional inequalities.

Of course, variations in the distribution of access, resources, and utilization in medical care are not a problem of only private-oriented systems. One reason for contrasting Britain with the United States in the following sections is to explore the distributional consequences of medical systems that are predominantly in the private sector with those which are more state dominated.

Although we do not focus on the causes of state intervention, we should note that a market-failures perspective can be used in order to understand why the state intervenes. Lack of access is an important market failure. When it is recognized, various classes pressure the state to remedy the unequal distribution of medical resources. The state responds to this political pressure with various programs designed to reduce inequality. The intentions behind state intervention, however, are not the same as its consequences. We must ask whether state intervention actually does equalize access and utilization.

We hypothesize that it does, for two reasons.[1] First, state intervention establishes hierarchical and bureaucratic systems that tend to emphasize standardization, routinization, and planning. For ease of management and administration, such systems are likely to comprise multiple levels of treatment, with standardized units at each level distributed according to cost-effectiveness (not the same thing as profitability). In France, Sweden, and, to a somewhat lesser extent, Britain, the delivery of medical services is intentionally organized around agglomerations of people, with hierarchies of specialized facilities serving large areas. The logic of state hierarchy tends to standardize administrative procedures and to reduce costs. Whatever the intentions of state bureaucrats, the result is the same: standardization of access, utilization, and (potentially) outcomes.

Second, state hierarchies tend to be dominated primarily by political, rather than economic considerations, and state officials are highly sensitive to political pressures. As belief in the efficacy of medical treatment has grown, political demands by lower-income groups have pushed central governments toward a distribution of resources which maximizes social and geographical equality.

Although state intervention may be expected to lead to greater equality in access to and distribution of medical resources, its effects on the utilization of medical services and on health outcomes are more ambiguous. The medical needs of low-income populations tend to be greater than those of upper-income groups for reasons of nutrition, occupation, style of life, and other risk factors (Townsend and Davidson, 1982). To relate consumption to needs, perfect equality of health outcomes would probably require a "reverse" inequality in which low-income groups would use far more medical resources than upper-income groups. Such utilization depends on belief in the efficacy of medical treatment, however, and on the quality of the experience for those receiving medical care. Even when access is equalized and resources are available, low-income populations may be less willing to seek medical care. They may well find it difficult to relate effectively to medical providers, who come from a different social class. The literature is filled with examples of how the social class backgrounds and life-styles of providers predispose them to be more responsive to clients of similar

1. The logic of markets has been much better developed by economists than the logic of hierarchy, especially state hierarchy. Lucien Karpik (1972b) has developed the idea of *logic d'active*, but this notion focuses primarily on the effort to develop coherent strategies in business corporations. Oliver E. Williamson (1975, 1985) and Alfred D. Chandler, Jr. (1977) have also used the idea of hierarchy to analyze the business corporation. Similar ideas need to be applied to political regimes and state hierachies. For an effort in this direction, see Lindblom 1977.

social backgrounds than to clients of lower income, class, and education. In other words, the treatment experience itself may be a disincentive for low-income consumers and an incentive for high-income consumers. Moreover, even if we assume equality of treatment across social groups, the medical needs of subpopulations vary substantially with social class and income levels, and available medical technologies are not equally efficacious for all types of health problems.

Some scholars believe that greater equality of access to and distribution of resources over a long period of time will promote greater equality of results. Others suggest that the outcomes of a single delivery system will not be substantially influenced by its institutional arrangements. Rather, the primary influence on equality of outcomes is the total structure and culture of a society. Even if a medical delivery system is egalitarian in access and distribution of resources, the outcomes will not be equal as long as inequality remains in the basic reward structure of the society—that is, income, occupational attainment, etc. (Bowles and Gintis, 1976; Jencks et al., 1972). In the sections that follow, we will be particularly sensitive to what the histories of the medical systems of the United States and Britain reveal about this debate. We hypothesize that state intervention will be far more effective in equalizing access and resource distribution then in equalizing outcomes.

Equality of Access

Differences between the British and American medical delivery systems in equality of access and historical changes within each system are clearly associated with medical specialization and state intervention. It is not possible to demonstrate the unique effects of medical specialization in limiting access to medical resources, because specialization and state intervention covary. Nevertheless, it is clear that a major effect of state intervention has been to increase equality in the access to medical services. In both nations, access has been enhanced as state intervention has increased, and the greater intervention of the British state is associated with wider access to medical resources.

In Britain, even before the introduction of the National Health Service in 1948, a number of state programs were already making medical care more accessible. First, the medical inspection of schoolchildren (introduced in 1907) had become sufficiently institutionalized by 1920 that every schoolchild in Britain was assured of at least three medical inspections before age fifteen. In most areas the local authorities would assume the cost of the child's treatment if parents were unable to pay (McCleary, 1933; *Political and Economic Planning*, 1937). Second, Parliament in 1918 urged the local authorities to provide maternity clinics and infant-welfare programs, with the result that by 1938, more than half of Britain's expectant mothers and infants received home visits and postnatal care (*Political and Economic Planning*, 1937). Third, the National Health Insurance system, introduced in 1912, provided outpatient medical care for ten million low-income working people who previously had not been covered by any form of medical insurance. Data on the extent of care are inexact, but certainly the system substantially increased access to care for those who were insured. By the 1930s, 77 percent of all men age fourteen to sixty-four, or approximately 40 percent of the total population, were covered (Titmuss, 1958; Levy, 1944). Fourth, the indigent and the elderly also received some medical care from the state, though the quality of care varied from place to place and over time. After the passage of the Old Age Pension Act in 1908, people eligible for old-age pensions also received medical assistance from Poor Law medical officers. Later, when various Poor Law facilities were abolished, the quality of public medical facilities and access to medical care improved for the indigent and elderly (Gilbert, 1966, 1970).

This patchwork of programs, although it doubtless improved access to medical care, also allowed considerable variation in services from place to place and group to group. Once the highly centralized National Health Service was introduced in 1948, however, everyone was entitled to the same service without any means tests or other restrictions (Stevens, 1966; Titmuss, 1958; Eckstein, 1958; Hollingsworth, 1986).

Although the long-term trend in American medical care has also been toward greater state intervention, and many government initiatives have improved access, government programs have not affected so large a portion of the society, nor have they formed a single coherent policy as in Britain. Instead, the state and federal governments engaged in a large number .of relatively small, categorical programs. These characterized the history of governmental efforts in the United States until the enactment of Medicare and Medicaid programs.

The involvement of the federal government in improving access to medical care was minimal prior to the 1920s. In that decade began a series of programs and subsidies aimed at the poor, children, mothers, and the disabled, as well as Native Americans, servicepeople, and veterans. Among the most important were the Sheppard Towner Act of 1922, the Federal Emergency Relief Administration (1933), Emergency Maternity and Infant Care Programs, and the Servicemen's Dependents Act (1956). Affecting access more substantially but less directly, the Hill-Burton Act of 1946 encouraged rapid growth in the number of available hospital beds. At various times, state and local governments have also provided medical assistance to the indigent.

Though the programs of the central, state, and local governments to increase equality of access have been numerous and expensive, they have not reached as large a portion of the population as the initiatives of the British state. Equality of access in the American health care system has increased but has not approached the level of the British system.

Geographical Distribution of Medical Resources

The unequal geographical distribution of medical resources has concerned medical policy makers in both nations. Medical resources under market-oriented conditions tend to become somewhat geographically concentrated as the complexity of medical specialization increases, and much state intervention has been designed to redistribute resources more equitably. As we would expect, Britain, with its greater level of state intervention, has been more successful than the United States in distributing medical care evenly throughout the country.

In Table 7.1, we present indexes of regional variation in the number of physicians and nurses, normed by the size of the population from 1890 to 1970. Because of data limitations, we focus on regions within England and Wales, not all of Great Britain. The really big changes in England and Wales, representing a 47 percent reduction of inequality in the regional distribution of physicians between 1951 and 1971, occurred after the introduction of the National Health Service in 1948.[2] In contrast, in the United States there was only a 12 percent reduction in regional imbalance. In Britain between 1951 and 1971, specialization increased only modestly, whereas it doubled in the U.S. One implication of these data is that the British state ensured better regional balance by preventing the spread of specialization as well as by balancing specialization across regions.

Similarly, in both Britain and the United States between 1950 and 1971 the regional imbalance in the distribution of nurses was reduced, but as one would expect, the reduction was much greater in England and Wales than in the United States, 76 percent versus 38 percent. In recent decades, the National Health Service in Britain appears to have enhanced the trend toward greater regional equality, whereas in the

2. A significant reduction in the regional variation of physicians between 1939 and 1941 was due to the mobilization of physicians in the armed services during the Second World War, as well as to state policy. For more extended analysis of these and related issues discussed in this chapter, see Hollingsworth 1986.

Table 7.1. Regional Distribution of Medical Personnel,
England and Wales and the United States, 1890–1971

| Year | Regional index $\left(\dfrac{\text{mean absolute deviation}}{\text{mean}} \times 100\right)$ | |
	Doctors per 100,000 population	Nurses per 100,000 population
	England and Wales	
1891	23.50	44.23
1901	21.06	39.18
1911	20.30	32.12
1921	23.80	34.12
1931	21.97	22.81
1941	12.42	13.76
1951	15.26	21.29
1961	11.15	11.42
1971	8.18	4.74
	United States	
1890	10.08	47.21
1900	12.49	35.60
1910	11.10	38.17
1920	9.46	34.82
1930	12.72	31.63
1940	18.84	28.84
1950	18.45	24.47
1960	17.33	15.34
1970	16.35	14.48

Sources: Britain, *Decennial Census*, 1891–1971; *U.S. Census*, 1890–1970.

United States increasing state intervention seems to have had little effect on the geographic distribution of medical personnel. In general, the American system has tended to promote specialization and maldistribution of resources, but the British system has tended to constrain specialization and facilitate greater equality.

The reasons for this pattern become clearer when the content of the programs in both nations is examined. In Britain under the National Health Insurance system (1912–1946), only outpatient care by general practitioners was covered. The system had little effect on the distribution of specialist practice, though this was indirectly affected by government subsidies for hospital construction and maintenance. Under the National Health Service, however, a system of "negative direction" was instituted, restricting the number of general practitioners in overdoctored areas. In addition, the National Health Service worked for a more even distribution of hospital beds across regions. These efforts were only partially successful in eliminating the regional inequalities that were built into the system during previous years, but they did move toward equalization.

Governmental programs in the United States have also been concerned with regional inequality but have been substantially less successful in reallocating medical facilities. Between 1940 and 1970, the period of greatest governmental activity, regional variation in the number of hospital beds and the number of admissions, both normed for population, remained roughly constant in the United States. Moreover, the impact of Medicaid throughout its history has been quite unequal across regions (Davis, 1975, 1976a, b). The American system had no mechanism like "negative direction" with which to allocate new facilities, nor did its methods of reimbursement to providers offer incentives to physicians to locate in less-wealthy or more sparsely populated areas. Indeed, the method of reimbursement has tended to encourage physicians to locate in more prosperous areas.

We must consider whether state intervention is the only way to distribute medical resources evenly throughout a country. Some have maintained that under market conditions, a convergence in the per capita income and wealth among regions will bring about the regional equalization of medical resources. In both the United States and Britain, however, regional per capita incomes have tended toward convergence. Nevertheless, medical resources have remained much more unevenly distributed in the United States (Schwartz et al., 1980). The more equitable regional distribution in the medical resources of Britain is probably attributable to the effects of greater state intervention, and the persisting inequalities of the American case are probably attributable to less state intervention and various market forces, including the greater specialization of the medical system in the United States.

Equality of Utilization

Even though equality of access and availability have been themes in the British and American systems, equalization of health outcomes is unlikely even when medical care is most efficacious unless resources are used proportionate to need. As medical systems grow more specialized and costs of treatment increase, equality of outcomes across income groups may decline unless steps are taken to equalize *effective* utilization of medical care.

The data in Tables 7.2 and 7.3 provide information on trends in physician utilization in the two countries. Table 7.2 gives the average number of consultations per year by income level or class before and after the introduction of the National Health Service. Inasmuch as the lowest-income group generally has more medical needs than the highest-income group, it is not surprising that in 1947, the year before the introduction of the National Health Service, the lowest-income group of males had 8.2 medical consultations, or 1.7 times as many as the highest-income group. Even so, one year after the introduction of the National Health Service, when medical care was available to everyone without a fee, the ratio of lowest- to highest-income group for both males and females increased substantially. In other words, when services were free to all, lower-income groups made even greater use of them.

There are no data on the consumption of medical care in England and Wales by income group after 1952, but the British have collected medical data by five social or occupational groupings, and with this data, it is possible to observe the consumption of medical care by five social classes for later dates. Social (or occupational) class I consists of higher professional and administrative occupations; class II of em-

Table 7.2. Average Annual Medical Consultations, by Income or Social Class, England and Wales, 1947–1971

Year	Sex and Age	Weekly earning levels					
		I More than £10	II £7–10	III £5–10	IV £5–7	V £3–5	VI Less than £3
		Consultations per person (ratio to level I)					
1947	Males, 16 and older	4.7 (1.0)	— —	4.1 (0.9)	— —	4.6 (1.0)	8.2 (1.7)
1947	Females, 16 and older	5.9 (1.0)	— —	5.0 (0.8)	— —	4.6 (0.8)	6.6 (1.1)
1949	Males, 16 and older	4.3 (1.0)	— —	4.1 (1.0)	— —	5.4 (1.3)	10.7 (2.5)
1949	Females, 16 and older	5.6 (1.0)	— —	5.3 (0.9)	— —	5.9 (1.1)	7.6 (1.4)
1951	Males, 21 and older	4.1 (1.0)	4.3 (1.0)	— —	4.9 (1.2)	7.1 (1.7)	9.2 (2.2)
1951	Females, 21 and older	4.7 (1.0)	5.3 (1.1)	— —	5.6 (1.2)	6.7 (1.4)	7.4 (1.6)
1952	Males and Females, 21 and older	3.1 (1.0)	4.1 (1.3)	— —	4.5 (1.4)	5.8 (1.9)	7.4 (2.4)

Table 7.2. (*Continued*)

Year	Sex and Age	Social class					
		I	II	IIIª	IIIᵇ	IV	V
		Consultations per person (ratio to class I)					
1955–56	Males, 15–64	2.2 (1.0)	2.5 (1.1)	3.1 (1.4)		3.4 (1.5)	3.7 (1.7)
1964	Males and Females, 16 and older	3.5 (1.0)	3.5 (1.0)	4.4 (1.3)	4.6 (1.3)	4.9 (1.4)	6.0 (1.7)
1970–71	Males, 15–64	2.7 (1.0)		2.6 (1.0)	2.9 (1.1)	3.5 (1.3)	
1970–71	Males, 15 and older	3.1 (1.0)		3.0 (1.0)	3.3 (1.1)	3.9 (1.3)	

Sources: Logan and Brooke, 1957:57; Rein, 1969:46; Great Britain, Office of Population Censuses and Surveys, Social Survey Division, 1973:319, 342.

Note: For 1947 and 1949 groups are classified according to the weekly income of the "chief wage earner" of a household, and for 1951 and 1952, according to the weekly income of the "head of the household." Consultation rates for 1947, 1949, and 1951 are estimated from published data on monthly rates per hundred persons. Data for the age groups 15–64 and 15 and older were calculated from published data on age groups 15–44, 45–64, and 65 and older, using sample populations as weights.

ªManual skilled occupations.

ᵇNonmanual skilled occupations.

ployers in industry and retail trades, as well as the lesser professions; class III skilled occupations; class IV, partly skilled occupations; and class V unskilled occupations. These data, also presented in Table 7.2, show for the period between 1955 and early 1971, the same pattern as the earlier data on medical consumption by income distribution: the National Health Service provided medical care somewhat in proportion to the level of individual need.[3]

In 1928–1931, the first period in which the consumption of medical services in the United States was systematically surveyed, less than half

3. One must be cautious not to overstate the degree of equality under the National Health Service. Several studies demonstrate that once one controls for need, lower occupational classes have fewer consultations than those in higher occupational groupings. Moreover, several studies have demonstrated that middle-class patients have longer consultations than lower-class patients. Moreover, middle-class patients are able to make better use of consultations, measured by the amount of information communicated, the number of communications, and the amount of knowledge doctors have of their middle-

of all Americans consulted a physician (see Table 7.3). And in 1963–1964, before the enactment of Medicare and Medicaid, the third of American families with the lowest income and the highest medical needs were less likely to consult physicians than those with higher incomes and fewer medical problems. After the enactment of Medicare and Medicaid, however, individuals with low incomes were more likely to consult physicians than those with higher incomes.

Table 7.3 reveals the striking changes that have occurred in access to medical care across income groups. In 1928–1931, individuals from the lowest-income group visited physicians less frequently than those with higher incomes, and in 1963–1964, the mean number of physician visits among the various income groups was almost the same. Following the introduction of Medicare and Medicaid, however, individuals in the lowest-income group, in greater need of medical care, visited physicians more frequently than individuals with higher incomes. The better access to medical facilities was especially marked among poor children, one-third of whom had not seen a physician for two years or more in 1964. By 1976, however, children from low-income families visited physicians as frequently as children in high-income families. And whereas only 58 percent of low-income women saw a physician early in pregnancy in 1963, that figure had changed to 71 percent in 1970 (Davis and Schoen, 1978:41–43).

And yet, serious inequities remained in the American system. For example, Medicare was designed to provide uniform medical benefits to all elderly persons covered by social security. But more than a decade after the enactment of the program, there were substantial differences in the use of medical services and in the receipt of Medicare payments, based on the income and race of recipients. Elderly persons with high incomes received twice the Medicare payments of individuals with low incomes. The average Medicare reimbursement for each physician visit was 50 percent more for high-income than for low-income persons, high-income individuals visited physicians almost 60 percent more frequently than low-income persons with similar health problems, and high-income individuals received 45 percent more days of hospital care than low-income individuals with similar health conditions (Davis and Schoen, 1978:92–119; Davis, 1975:449–88). Part of this differential in Medicare benefits resulted from the greater likelihood that upper-income individuals would seek out specialists, whose practices were

class patients (Cartwright and O'Brien, 1976; Cartwright, 1964; Townsend and Davidson, 1982). And whereas family planning, maternity, and a variety of other preventive services are available to all, other studies have demonstrated that the manual occupational classes make considerably less use of them than those higher in the occupational scale (Townsend and Davidson, 1982).

Table 7.3. Consulting Physicians and Mean Number of Physician Visits per Year, by Family Income, United States, 1928–1976

| | | Income group* | | |
		High	Medium	Low
1928–1931	Percentage consulting physician	53	47	44
(whites only)	Ratio to high-income group	1.0	.89	.83
	Mean number of physician visits	3.1	2.2	2.0
	Ratio to high-income group	1.0	.71	.65
1963–1964	Percentage consulting physician	72	64	56
	Ratio to high-income group	1.0	.90	.79
	Mean number of physician visits	4.6	4.3	4.4
	Ratio to high-income group	1.0	.93	.96
1970	Percentage consulting physician	71	67	65
	Ratio to high-income group	1.0	.94	.92
	Mean number of physician visits	3.6	3.9	4.9
	Ratio to high-income group	1.0	1.08	1.36
1976	Percentage consulting physician	79	75	73
	Ratio to high-income group	1.0	.94	.92
	Mean number of physician visits	3.8	4.0	4.6
	Ratio to high-income group	1.0	1.05	1.21

Sources: Falk et al., 1933:110; Andersen et al., 1976:48; Aday, et al., 1980.

*For each time point, approximately one-third of the families surveyed were in each of the three income groups.

in high-income areas and who were staff members in high-image hospitals, whereas low-income people tended to gravitate more frequently to general practitioners whose practices were in low-income neighborhoods. And the low-income person was more likely to visit an emergency clinic or to be hospitalized in a large, crowded public general hospital.

While Medicare guidelines scrupulously specified that services were to be available to the elderly without discrimination, black Americans tended to receive fewer services than white Americans, even though blacks tended to have more serious health problems. For example, whites in the late 1960s received 60 percent more benefits for physician services than blacks under Medicare, and more than double the benefits for skilled-nursing services. In general, blacks tended to receive more of their Medicare services from less-specialized physicians and hospital outpatient departments; this care was more fragmented and impersonal than that received by whites, who had greater access to private physicians (Davis, 1975).

The greatest inequity in the Medicaid program was that people in the same circumstances were not treated the same in all parts of the country. The eligibility requirements for Medicaid vary substantially from state to state. By 1975 at least eight million poor people were ex-

cluded from Medicaid coverage, and some studies, adjusting for the
large number of people moving in and out of Medicaid over time, suggest that as much as 40 percent of the poor population was not covered
at any given time (Davis, 1976a:313). In 1969 Medicaid payments were
75 percent higher for white than for black recipients, partly because
more blacks were concentrated in the South, where Medicaid programs
were very limited. Even in the northeastern states, however, whites
received almost 50 percent more Medicaid benefits than blacks (Davis,
1976a:314). Clearly Medicaid did not achieve the goals of providing all
citizens with the best medical practice the country possessed. Many
physicians were reluctant to participate in the program because Medicaid reimbursed at lower rates than private insurance companies.
Other disincentives to physician participation included the cumber-
some bureaucracy of the program, payment delays, and restrictions on
the type of services covered (Davis, 1976a:316).

Despite programs for the indigent, the poor and the nonpoor were
clearly receiving very different types of medical care throughout the
1970s. Care for poor people was usually fragmented, impersonal, and
episodic, administered mainly in crowded, even dirty clinics with long
waits and few amenities. Few poor children received care from pedi-
atricians, and high-income women by 1970 were twice as likely to be
cared for by a specialist as poor women (Davis, 1976b). The poor tended to spend 50 percent more time than the nonpoor in traveling and
waiting to see a physician. Moreover, persons with incomes below three
thousand dollars in the early 1970s were spending essentially the same
fraction of their income on medical care as in 1963—before Medicaid
and Medicare came into existence. Persons with incomes below two
thousand dollars spent an average of almost 15 percent of their income
for medical services (Davis and Schoen, 1978).

It appears that state intervention in Britain has resulted in one-fifth
more utilization of the medical system by the working class than by
upper-income groups. If we assume that the medical needs of the poor
are approximately the same in Britain and the United States, we can
conclude with some confidence that greater state intervention in the
British system substantially contributed to a closer fit between need and
utilization than was the case in the United States. Furthermore, increasing governmental intervention in both nations has clearly enhanced the
ability of the poor to obtain medical care.

Equality of Results: Levels of Health

Although many believe that medical treatment has become much more
efficacious in recent decades, equality in utilization of medical services

does not guarantee equality in levels of health across social classes and income groups. Many of the "nonmedical" factors that affect health are unequally distributed. Despite improvements, mortality rates in both countries still vary according to region and social class.[4]

To some extent the data for England and Wales in Table 7.4 support the hypothesis that equality in the distribution of medical resources leads to equality of results. Greater state intervention, which distributes medical resources more equitably throughout all regions, appears to reduce regional variation in levels of health. For almost every age category, regional variation in mortality declined following the introduction of the National Health Service. Regional variation in infant mortality increased in England and Wales between 1891 and 1931, but between 1931 and 1971 it declined substantially. Those age twenty-four to forty-four followed the same pattern. Among those age forty-five to sixty-four, most of the decline in regional variation occurred after the introduction of the National Health Service, although it had begun earlier. Similarly, the decline in the regional variation in age-sex standardized death rates, modest but steady for sixty years, accelerated after 1951.

These data, however, will not permit the conclusion that more equitable regional distribution of medical resources caused levels of health in various regions to converge. The relationship may well be spurious. Since the late nineteenth century, regional variation in per capita income and standard of living has also decreased. Quite possibly this factor was responsible for the data in Table 7.4.

Fortunately, data on the United States provide some insight. In the more market-oriented system of the United States regional variation in the distribution of medical resources has diminished very little, but regional variations in mortality have declined, in association with variability in regional per capita income. Most likely, the greater uniformity in standard of living from one region to the other, particularly in the United States, is primarily responsible for reduced variation in regional mortality rates.

Comparisons of levels of health across social classes are somewhat less problematic, in that income differences among social classes have generally declined much less than among regions. Moreover, infant mortality rates offer a telling and sensitive index of health differences between social classes because of the demonstrable connection between improvements in medical technology and their decline. In Tables 7.5 and 7.6, we present neonatal (first month), postneonatal (months 2–12), and infant mortality (sum of deaths in the first year) rates by the

4. Again, we note that mortality rates—though not as refined a measure of health as morbidity, disability, and illness rates—are the only data available in both countries throughout the period.

Table 7.4. Index of Regional Variation in Mortality Rates, the United States and England and Wales, 1890–1970

	1890–1891	1900–1901	1910–1911	1920–1921	1930–1931	1940–1941	1950–1951	1960–1961	1970–1971
				Regional index $\left(\dfrac{\text{mean absolute deviation}}{\text{mean}} \times 100\right)$					
All persons age 0–1									
England and Wales	8.1	9.6	9.6	13.9	14.7	NA	13.9	7.1	6.9
United States, white	26.9	12.9	19.4	13.2	9.6	13.9	11.8	6.6	5.5
United States, nonwhite	39.3	30.9	33.3	21.6	18.6	10.6	19.3	11.2	9.0
United States, total	26.6	25.0	21.7	12.2	10.8	17.8	15.8	12.2	9.7
All persons age 25–44									
England and Wales	11.6	8.0	9.2	9.5	12.4	NA	12.6	11.1	7.8
United States, white	6.2	10.7	10.1	7.3	8.5	8.6	8.0	6.9	8.0
United States, nonwhite	8.9	10.4	18.8	7.0	10.4	11.5	12.1	11.8	14.0
United States, total	5.7	15.0	12.4	13.3	18.8	17.1	15.3	12.1	11.9
All persons age 45–64									
England and Wales	11.0	9.1	9.1	8.5	8.5	NA	10.2	8.0	6.9
United States, white	12.0	13.9	11.1	7.9	7.8	7.3	7.4	5.1	4.0
United States, nonwhite	14.5	10.6	20.2	10.8	13.0	13.0	15.0	13.4	13.7
United States, total	11.9	17.2	12.2	8.2	9.1	8.4	7.7	6.2	7.3
*All persons, age-sex standardized population**									
England and Wales	9.3	8.4	7.9	8.1	8.9	NA	8.2	6.4	5.4
United States, white	9.1	8.8	10.4	5.9	5.2	3.2	3.3	3.1	2.6
United States, nonwhite	17.7	13.6	27.3	8.8	8.1	7.1	8.8	7.4	10.7
United States, total	10.8	14.1	12.0	5.7	7.0	5.3	4.8	4.2	4.3

Sources: Great Britain, *Decennial Census*, 1891–1971; Great Britain, *Registrar General Reports*, 1891–1971; *Vital Statistics of the United States* (Annual Reports).

*Standardized on the population of England and Wales, 1931.

Table 7.5. Neonatal and Postneonatal Mortality, by Social Class, England and Wales, 1911–1972

Year	Social class I	Social class II	Social class III*		Social class IV	Social class V
			Deaths per 1,000 births (ratio to rate of class I)			
			Neonatal			
1911	30.26 (1.0)	36.5 (1.2)	36.8 (1.2)		38.6 (1.3)	42.5 (1.4)
1921	23.4 (1.0)	28.3 (1.2)	33.7 (1.4)		36.7 (1.6)	36.9 (1.6)
1930–1932	21.7 (1.0)	27.2 (1.3)	29.4 (1.4)		31.9 (1.5)	32.5 (1.5)
1939	18.9 (1.0)	23.4 (1.2)	25.4 (1.3)		27.7 (1.5)	30.1 (1.6)
1950	12.9 (1.0)	16.2 (1.3)	17.6 (1.4)		19.8 (1.5)	21.9 (1.7)
1964–1965	9.2 (1.0)		11.8 (1.3)		13.2 (1.4)	
1970–1972 Males	8.9 (1.0)	9.7 (1.1)	10.7 (1.2)	11.0 (1.2)	12.7 (1.4)	17.0 (1.9)
Females	6.3 (1.0)	7.4 (1.2)	7.6 (1.2)	8.2 (1.3)	9.1 (1.4)	17.6 (2.0)
			Postneonatal			
1911	46.2 (1.0)	69.9 (1.5)	75.9 (1.6)		82.9 (1.8)	110.0 (2.4)
1921	15.0 (1.0)	27.2 (1.8)	43.1 (2.8)		52.7 (3.5)	60.1 (4.0)
1930–1932	11.0 (1.0)	17.8 (1.6)	28.2 (2.6)		34.9 (3.2)	44.6 (4.1)
1939	7.9 (1.0)	11.0 (1.4)	19.0 (2.4)		23.7 (3.0)	30.0 (3.8)
1950	4.9 (1.0)	6.0 (1.2)	10.5 (2.1)		13.9 (2.8)	18.8 (3.8)
1964–1965	3.5 (1.0)		5.4 (1.5)		7.6 (2.2)	
1970–1972 Males	3.5 (1.0)	4.1 (1.2)	4.6 (1.3)	6.2 (1.8)	7.3 (2.1)	14.6 (4.2)
Females	2.3 (1.0)	3.2 (1.4)	3.1 (1.3)	5.0 (2.2)	6.0 (2.6)	11.6 (5.1)

Sources: Titmuss, 1943:37; Great Britain, Registrar General, 1938, 1954:24; Spicer and Lipworth, 1966:21, 26; Great Britain, Office of Population Censuses and Surveys, 1978:157.

*For 1970–1972, class III is divided into nonmanual and manual skilled occupations, respectively.

Table 7.6. Infant Mortality by Social Class, England and Wales, 1911–1972

Year	Deaths per 1,000 births (ratio to rate of class I)				
	Social class I	Social class II	Social class III[a]	Social class IV	Social class V
1899[b]	94 (1.0)	— —	173 (1.8)	184 (2.0)	247 (2.6)
1911	76 (1.0)	106 (1.4)	113 (1.5)	122 (1.6)	153 (2.0)
1921–1923	38 (1.0)	55 (1.4)	77 (2.0)	89 (2.3)	97 (2.6)
1930–1932	33 (1.0)	45 (1.4)	58 (1.8)	67 (2.0)	77 (2.3)
1939	27 (1.0)	34 (1.3)	44 (1.6)	51 (1.9)	60 (2.2)
1949–1953	19 (1.0)	22 (1.2)	29 (1.5)	34 (1.8)	41 (2.2)
1964–1965	12.7 (1.0)		17.2 (1.4)	20.8 (1.6)	
1970–1972	12 (1.0)	14 (1.2)	15 (1.3) 17 (1.4)	(1.7)	(2.6)

Sources: Great Britain, Office of Population Censuses and Surveys 1978:182; Great Britain, Registrar General, 1923, 1927, 1938; United Nations, 1954; Parker et al., 1972; Rowntree, 1908:198–208.

[a]For 1970–1972, the two categories of social class III data refer to nonmanual skilled and manual skilled occupations, respectively.

[b]For 1899, data refer to the servant-keeping class of York and to selected districts in York coded by Rowntree (1908) according to the proportion of families living in primary and secondary poverty as determined by a comparison of family income and minimum budgets. Rowntree defined primary poverty by family income insufficient to purchase the physical necessities of life. Families in secondary poverty could potentially afford necessities, though in fact a portion of their income was absorbed by "useless or wasteful" expenditures. The population of Rowntree's area A consisted of 6,803 people (1,642 families) of whom 70 percent lived in primary or secondary poverty; 37 percent of the 9,945 inhabitants of area B lived in primary or secondary poverty. None of the 5,336 people in area C lived in primary or secondary poverty. In this table, area A data is coded as class V, area B data as class IV, area C data as class III, and the servant-keeping class as class I.

occupation of the father in England and Wales for the period between 1899 and 1982. Improved standards of living and developments in medical practice have dramatically reduced all components of infant mortality, especially postneonatal death rates. Even more striking, however, is that differences among classes have remained essentially constant, despite substantial equalization in access to and utilization of medical resources.

There are a number of reasons for this persistence. Providing medical services from public revenues does not necessarily ensure effective use of the system. People must know when to visit the physician, and if they misjudge, the consequences can be very serious. Obviously, the better educated and the better informed can use the system more ad-

Table 7.7. Neonatal and Postneonatal, and Infant Mortality, by Income Level, United States, 1911–1966

Year	Deaths per 1,000 births (ratio to rate of level I)				
	Income level I	Income level II	Income level III	Income level IV	Income level V
Neonatal					
1911–1916	36.6 (1.00)	41.3 (1.13)	46.0 (1.26)	44.6 (1.22)	54.2 (1.48)
1964–1966	18.5 (1.00)	17.1 (0.93)	16.8 (0.91)	22.4 (1.21)	30.2 (1.63)
Postneonatal					
1911–1916	27.5 (1.00)	50.2 (1.83)	62.9 (2.29)	76.7 (2.78)	107.8 (3.92)
1964–1966	3.9 (1.00)	4.9 (1.25)	5.1 (1.30)	8.5 (2.14)	15.1 (3.83)
Infant					
1911–1916	64.0 (1.00)	91.5 (1.43)	108.7 (1.70)	120.8 (1.89)	162.0 (2.53)
1964–1966	22.4 (1.00)	22.0 (0.98)	21.9 (0.98)	30.0 (1.38)	45.3 (2.02)

Sources: Woodbury, 1925:148–51; National Center for Health Statistics, Computer Tape of the National Infant Mortality and National Mortality Survey, 1972.

Notes: Data for 1911–1916 refer to all births and postneonatal deaths in seven cities, each surveyed for twelve consecutive months between 1911 and 1916. The cities were Baltimore, Maryland; New Bedford and Brockton, Massachusetts; Waterbury, Connecticut; Manchester, New Hampshire; Akron, Ohio; and Saginaw, Michigan. The data have been reanalyzed for this table. Data for 1964–1966 are based on a national probability sample of legitimate and illegitimate births.

vantageously. And these people are more apt to seek out better doctors and better hospitals.

For the United States, the data are more fragmentary (see Table 7.7). These limited observations are based on income rather than occupation, and for the 1911–1916 period, the data refer to only seven cities. Despite these deficiencies, the table reveals a similar dramatic improvement in overall rates of mortality and a similar lack of marked change in the differential life chances of social groups. Very revealing for the United States are the more complete data on white and nonwhite infant mortality contained in Table 7.8. Again, we see great overall improvement in both groups but no narrowing of differentials between the two groups until the most recent period (1964–1975). Since white-black income differentials have remained substantial, we believe that the narrowing of these infant mortality differentials is due to the impact of Medicaid and other government programs.

Data on the mortality of adult women by social class or income group are extremely limited. Classifying women according to the occupational group of their husbands, mortality rate differentials declined slightly in

Table 7.8. White and Nonwhite Neonatal,
Postneonatal, and Infant Mortality Rates,
United States, 1925–1975

Year	Deaths per 1,000 births		Ratio of nonwhite to white
	White	Nonwhite	
Neonatal			
1925	36.8	49.5	1.35
1950	19.4	27.5	1.41
1960	17.2	26.9	1.56
1964	16.2	26.5	1.65
1975	10.7	15.8	1.47
Postneonatal			
1925	31.5	61.3	1.95
1950	7.4	17.0	2.30
1960	5.7	16.3	2.86
1964	5.4	14.6	2.70
1975	3.7	7.1	1.92
Infant			
1925	68.3	110.8	1.62
1950	26.8	44.5	1.66
1960	22.9	43.2	1.88
1964	21.5	41.4	1.92
1975	14.4	22.9	1.59

Source: Grove and Hetzel, 1968.

England and Wales between 1930 and 1950 and appear to have widened somewhat since that time (Hollingsworth, 1979:22), as have deaths of mothers at childbirth. Data on women by income group and social class in the United States are largely unavailable, but some comparisons between white and nonwhite women are possible (U.S. Census Office, 1975; Grove and Hetzel, 1968:330–33). These data show results similar to those in England and Wales. Overall, the differential (age-adjusted) in mortality rates of white and nonwhite women narrowed very little between 1920 and 1970. In fact, the gap in maternal mortality increased markedly from 1920 to 1970 (nonwhites were 1.7 times more likely to die in 1920 and 4.0 times more likely by 1970).

Data for American adult males comparable to those compiled by the registrar general in Britain do not exist for all years, but there are enough data to observe that the pattern in the United States has resembled that in England and Wales. Among white males in the United States between 1950 and 1960, inequality widened just as it did in England and Wales during the same period. On the other hand, the gap between white and nonwhite males was narrowing. In 1900 the morality ratio between the highest and lowest occupational groups was wider in England and Wales than in the United States, but by 1950 the gap between these groups was less in England and Wales than in the United States. In 1960 the gap between the two groups was about the same in England and Wales as it was for white American males, though if one considers both nonwhites and whites, there was greater inequality in health in the United States than in England and Wales. And this is a major point. According to the data, state intervention has not reduced regional inequality of outcomes in Britain, but it does seem to be associated with greater equality among occupational groupings (Great Britain, Office of Population Censuses and Surveys, 1978:174; Great Britain, Registrar General, 1891–1971; U.S. Census Office, 1896, 1900; Kitagawa and Hauser, 1973).

Clearly, Western nations have not yet equalized the chances for good health in all regions and for people of all races, income levels, and social classes. From a policy perspective, one may regard the glass as being either half empty or half full. In both the United States and Britain, increased state intervention has brought increased equality, and the greater the intervention, the greater is the equality of access, resource allocation, and utilization. On the other hand, we have uncovered far less evidence that equality of medical care results in equality of health.

The data we have offered support our general hypothesis that increasing specialization and differentiation of medical treatment may in themselves lead to greater inequality. As the unit cost of medical care increases and medical technology becomes more specialized and interdependent, geographical and social inequalities are intensified.

State intervention provides one means of adjusting for this tendency, to maintain or increase the equality of access to and distribution of medical resources. One form of state intervention, the American approach, is to subsidize the costs of medical care so that more citizens—especially the poor—can afford medical care. Another form of state intervention, the British approach, is to provide care directly, removing most medical services from the market.

One of the most important findings of our investigation is that equal opportunity does not translate automatically into equal results. In the medical area (as in education, housing, transportation, and other areas of social policy), unequal results are, to a substantial degree, determined by general patterns of societal inequality. As long as income, wealth, housing, education, and other important resources are unevenly distributed, levels of health are likely to reflect these inequalities. Nevertheless, state-sponsored compensatory programs can reduce inequality, even if they cannot eliminate it.

8

STATE INTERVENTION
VERSUS PRIVATIZATION

Each national medical system is a unique product of the specific cultural, political, legal, and social environment of the society in which it is located. Partly for this reason, most literature on national medical systems focuses on system idiosyncracies, or specific policies in particular nations. It is more descriptive than theoretical. This viewpoint, though rewarding, has limitations for policy analysis. In this book, therefore, we have undertaken a broader perspective, studying national medical systems in a comparative and historical framework and at a more theoretical level. This approach provides us with somewhat different insights about the nature of the problems confronting Western medical systems and the debates surrounding proposals for reform. By examining how differing nations deal with similar problems (for example, high costs and complex technologies), we believe we can better understand the importance of institutional arrangements, especially the consequences of state intervention and investments in human capital and medical technology.

The Debate over Privatization

Over the years since 1890 each of the four medical systems has encountered a series of performance "crises," which have often led to substantial institutional changes, especially state intervention. In the 1980s the "crisis" has involved uncontrollable increases in costs, driven by rapid progress in medical technology and rising popular demand for services. Every nation has formulated policies designed to limit costs while maintaining adequate performance along other dimensions. Recently, some analysts have maintained that state intervention is a major cause of current difficulties, and they have proposed privatization as a means of addressing poor performance of national medical systems. The exact meaning of *privatization* is far from clear (Starr, 1987), but most variants call for radical reductions in what we have called state intervention.

To understand the debate about privatization, it is useful to study the history of the development of medical care. During the course of economic development and "modernization," medical technology has become more complex and expensive, the number of medical personnel has increased greatly, the public has developed high expectations about the efficaciousness of medical technology, and people live longer and place increasing demands on the system.

As the economies of Western Europe and North America rapidly expanded after World War II, the state became substantially more involved in financing medical care, resulting in a marked shift toward increased consumption and greater equity in utilization. In France, Great Britain, and the United States, professional providers were vigorously opposed to increased state intervention—especially when it posed a potential threat to professional autonomy. Their powerful influence made it difficult for the state to move out of the realm of finance to begin manipulating the supply of medical care. In most countries, a fundamental compromise was struck. Physicians accepted public funding to subsidize system expansion but insisted on continued control over the pricing and allocation of care. State managers and politicians, faced with increasing popular pressure for service expansion, were often willing to accommodate provider's demands in an era of generally rapid economic growth. Not only did physicians retain their autonomy, but in most countries their relative incomes increased substantially as a result of their compromise with the state.

In most countries this very costly arrangement was tolerable as long as economic growth was substantial. Once growth slowed or stopped, however, the compromise between physicians and the state became more troublesome. More and more of the society's resources were spent on medical care. Thus, the capacity of the state to fund services declined, while demand for services and development of expensive medical technology increased, making the cost of medical care a salient political issue. In an effort to contain spending, nations have begun to consider state coordination and regulation of the supply side of medical care. With this proposal, the compromise that made medical welfare services possible begins to break down. In one country, then another, medical providers have begun to call for the privatization of medical care (Manga and Weller, 1980; Weller and Manga, 1983; Hollingsworth, 1986).

The costs of medical care and the goals of providers are not the only considerations in the debate over privatization. Other possible goals include improvements in health, development of new technologies, equitable access to medical services, and reasonable costs for consumers. It is extraordinarily difficult to achieve all these goals simultaneously. Yet groups concerned with one or another of these goals often call for more or less state regulation as a means of achieving their preferred ends. We might have concerned ourselves with how these pressures have influenced institutional arrangements. Instead, however, we wanted to see what effects the arrangements themselves have had on such variables as costs, levels of health, innovativeness, social efficiency, and equality. In the wide-ranging debate about the desired institutional forms, it is well to know exactly what results each variation, from completely privatized to completely state controlled, might be expected to produce. Nevertheless, in this last chapter we also want to define the actors in the debate and to be sensitive to their preferences. The debate over privatization is taking place along the lines depicted in Figure 8.1, though the specific proposals, the intensity of debate, and the groups involved vary somewhat from country to country.

Most research on interest groups has been idiosyncratic, focusing on specific issues within a single country, rather than looking for common themes at different times and in different countries. On the basis of extensive reading, we believe that it is possible to develop a general scheme of interest groups and policy outcomes that applies to most industrialized countries. Historically, such groups have been critical in shaping system performance by their influence on institutional arrangements, and three major groups have always been relevant: consumers, providers (that is, physicians and hospital administrators), and government officials. Consumers are usefully subdivided into two income groups whose interests frequently diverge. Obviously, each of these groups is internally heterogeneous, and such broad categories would oversimplify a study of a particular piece of legislation or a single administrative decision. For the purposes of understanding decisions about investment in medical care, access to and allocation and location of resources, and the readiness of systems to adopt various types of structural change, however, this approach is sufficient.

Figure 8.1 diagrams the preferences of major interest groups.

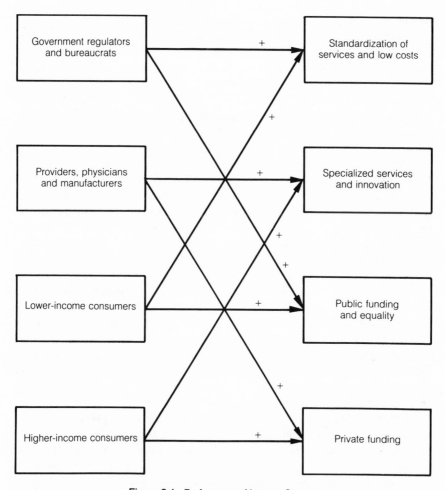

Figure 8.1. Preferences of Interest Groups

Lower-income consumers have been most interested in equalizing access to care and benefits via public spending and in promoting general services, rather than highly specialized ones. Upper-income groups have sought highly individualized and differentiated services. Historically they have been much more concerned than lower-income consumers with innovations, and they have promoted medical research and specialized personal services. Upper-income groups have tended to prefer goods provided in the private sector, for privatized systems permit more prosperous individuals to influence the form, quantity, and utilization of medical services.

Professional providers have seen programmatic and technological innovations as important, largely because these have called for more development of their special skills and have tended to enhance their incomes and prestige. Similarly, professional providers have promoted specialized services, which in turn have stimulated technical innovations. Because professional providers have preferred the type of organization into which they have been socialized, they have been less inclined to support organizational innovations, even though the technical innovations they supported have often led to new types of organizations.

Whereas professional organizations have often opposed organizational and technological standardization for fear of losing control over services, government administrators have tended to favor standardization as a means of reducing costs and maintaining accountability in public programs. For the same reason they have been less supportive of technical innovations. Government officials are desirous of legitimating systems by coordinating the interests of other groups, and as the size of national medical systems has expanded, government officials have acquired more autonomy and have had more opportunity to shape the system.

Potentially, several natural coalitions exist in this pattern. Lower-income groups and government bureaucrats tend to prefer the same benefits; providers and higher-income groups tend to agree on other preferences. The exact lines of coalition among interest groups have varied from country to country, but the basic distinctions have been those of Figure 8.1.

In all four countries, providers have been the most powerful group and have done more than any other group to shape system structure and processes, but their power has varied from country to country. In some, it has been counterbalanced by relatively influential lower-income groups and government bureaucrats. The issue of privatization has emerged in all four countries, but its advocates have had the boldest designs in those countries where providers have enjoyed the most power (for a fuller discussion, see Hage and Hollingsworth, 1977; Hollingsworth and Hanneman, 1984; Hollingsworth, 1986; Alford, 1975; Abel-Smith, 1965; Hogarth, 1963; Klein, 1983).

The most vocal advocates of privatization in the United States have been medical providers, though they have been joined by business leaders, scholars in research organizations, the insurance industry, and leaders of the Republican party. In Britain the leadership has come from elements within the British Medical Association, assisted by ideologues in the Conservative party and elements in the insurance industry. The support for privatization in France and Sweden has been somewhat more narrowly based, the most articulate spokespersons being medical providers. The particular terms of the debate have likewise varied somewhat from country to country. For example, in the United States advocates of privatization have had little sympathy for universal entitlements to state-financed services, whereas in Sweden universal entitlements are taken for granted. On the other hand, in all countries advocates of privatization wish to shift some of the financial responsibility for medical care from the state to individuals via private insurance schemes. Advocates of privatization argue that market forces should become more prominent in the delivery of medical services, though what is meant by market forces varies. In all four countries, advocates of privatization argue for coinsurance, deductibles, and the expansion of private medical insurance. In the United States, advocates of privatization believe that coinsurance and deductibles will help to constrain rising medical costs. In Great Britain, however, where many are convinced that the state has underfunded the medical system, advocates believe that private medical insurance will increase the level of spending on medical care and raise the income of medical providers.

In other words, privatization is viewed in some countries as a means of bringing about cost containment and utilization restriction, while in other societies it is meant to have the opposite effect. In all countries, however, advocates of privatization see the expansion of the private sector as a means of reducing tax rates, lowering public spending, balancing state budgets, curbing the growth in the state sector, and enhancing flexibility in the delivery of medical services.

Empirical Analysis

We have attempted to bring empirical analysis to bear on issues relevant to this debate. Specifically, we have endeavored to measure the impact of state-sector coordinating mechanisms on the performance of national medical systems. To measure the impact of state intervention on system performance systematically we developed a research design that included services provided by both private and government sectors. Moreover, we recognized that in the state sector there has been more than one type of control and that the consequences for performance have varied with different types of control. From reading widely in the medical histories of various countries, we became convinced not only that centralization is a critical variable shaping system performance but also that the least centralized system is that in which all decisions over finance, pricing, and personnel are made in the private sector. In a somewhat more centralized system all decisions are made in the public sector, but by local or regional authorities. The most centralized systems are those in which all decisions are controlled by the central government.

In Table 8.1, we summarize the results of our analysis, both qualitative and quantitative, for as we have emphasized, given the complexity of the problem, we must concern ourselves with a variety of evidence. In this table we also indicate whether the direct and net effects of the quantitative data are the same. To simplify the discussion, we report only the direction of the relationship.

In the first line, for example, we report whether state control over prices and personnel influences the costs of medical care. The results demonstrate that state intervention in the delivery of medical care has consequences contrary to what many proponents of privatization have argued, but the consequences of the two dimensions of state intervention are not identical for each performance measure. In general, the quantitative evidence about medical costs is somewhat stronger for control over prices and personnel than it is for control over revenues. If the state is only involved in funding medical care but does *not* control prices and appoint personnel, medical prices tend to be higher and to increase more rapidly than if the state both funds medical care *and* controls prices and appoints personnel.

The impact of the two state-intervention variables on levels of health

Table 8.1. Assessment of State Intervention in Medical Systems

Performance	Control over revenues			Control over prices and personnel		
	Direct path coefficients	Net effects	Qualitative assessment	Direct path coefficients	Net effects	Qualitative assessment
Costs	+	Nil[a]	+	−	−	−
Mortality	+	−	−	−	−	−
Social efficiency	−	Nil[a]	−	+	+	+
Innovativeness Diffusion time of immunizations*	−	−	−	−	−	−
	Qualitative assessments					
	Control over revenues			Control over prices and personnel		
Innovativeness Diffusion time of high-cost technologies	−			+		
Equality Access to care	+			+		
Regional equalization of services	+			+		

*Based on data presented in Figure 5.2.

[a]Nil effect is defined as ≤ .05.

is similar, and both variables contribute to the decline in age-sex standardized mortality rates. The one qualification is the direct effect of state control of revenues on mortality. For us, however, the more critical findings are the total net effects and the considerable qualitative evidence presented in Chapter 4, which indicate that control over revenues improves access to care and thus reduces a society's mortality. These findings are important, for many people assume that the quality of medical services is higher in the private than the public sector. Yet even if some of the world's best medical service is in the private sector, in the aggregate the mortality rates of entire societies are more likely to be reduced by state intervention. Perhaps the most critical finding is that as the state increases its control over both prices and personnel, mortality is reduced even further. These findings which are quite robust, demonstrate that state mechanisms of coordination and control can improve the level of health in a society.

Increases in state funding of medical services does result in more expensive medical systems, as those advocating privatization have claimed. But another important consequence of state control over revenues should not be overlooked. Historically, state funding leads to state involvement in many other aspects of medical delivery systems and eventually to greater control over prices and personnel. In the United States, for example, the financing of medical care for the elderly under the Medicare program contributed to a dramatic increase in medical spending, so that the federal government responded in 1983 with the diagnostic related groupings (DRG) program in an effort to regulate expenditures for hospital services. Such increases in state control over prices and personnel in all four countries have slowed the rise in medical expenditures.

The biggest benefit of state control over prices and personnel is in the area where the proponents of privatization have expressed their greatest concern: the problem of social efficiency. We find that state financing of medical care is counterproductive relative to social efficiency. The increased costs that directly result from state funding are not compensated by sizable reductions in mortality. State control over prices and personnel, however, improves the trade-off between mortality reduction and cost escalation, resulting in greater social efficiency.

The relationship between state intervention and innovativeness was rather complex. We analyzed various low-priced innovations desired by most everyone and more expensive innovations desired by only a small proportion of the population. We also studied the speed with which innovations were first adopted and the speed with which they diffused throughout a national system. Our research indicated that once immunizations (low-priced innovations) were demonstrated to be relatively safe and efficacious, state intervention had little effect on the interval before adoption, which was brief in all countries. On the other hand, the analysis demonstrated that centralized state intervention led to a faster diffusion of vaccines throughout the system. With regard to new drugs, state centralization slowed adoption, and expensive innovations demanded by relatively small groups also tended to diffuse more slowly throughout nations with more centralized systems.

Low-income consumer support for increased state intervention is often based on the belief that state-coordinated systems distribute medical care more equitably than privately coordinated ones. Our analysis confirms this belief. In the systems for which we have data, increasing state coordination of medical services increases the equality in access to care and the volume of services available and reduces inequality in the regional distribution of medical resources. State coordination, however, has not tended to reduce inequality in levels of health across social classes and income groups. The degree of variation in health status appears to be influenced more by the way income, education, and lifestyles vary than by the way medical resources are distributed.

The Logic of Privatization and State Intervention

In the first chapter, we suggested the need for a new direction in institutional analysis, and in subsequent chapters, we concentrated on the consequences of various institutional arrangements. We must also confront the problem of myths, a theme in institutional analysis (Meyer and Rowan, 1977). The myths that privatization helps to reduce total costs and that competitiveness and private orientation improve the efficiency of medical care are widely shared but, as our analysis demonstrates, not supported by the data. Clearly, privatization in the delivery of medical care does not have the advantages its proponents claim for it, but why? We are led to another critical issue in institutional analysis—what might be called the logic of various kinds of institutional arrangements.

Exploring the logic of privatization and state intervention can, we hope, help to explain the reasons for the relationships outlined in Table 8.1 and can contribute to the growing literature in institutional analysis (Zucker, 1987; Scott, 1987). As we suggested in Chapter 3 physicians are more dominant over ambulatory and hospital care the more the medical system is privatized. Theirs is the most powerful interest involved in the delivery of medical care, and a high level of privatization, therefore, leads to higher levels of consumption, duplication of expensive equipment (especially in urban contexts), higher costs, and lower efficiency. Furthermore, better-educated physicians prefer urban contexts, so that there is a strong concentration of medical resources in urban areas, with relatively few resources in rural areas.

We have suggested several reasons why patients, unlike other consumers, cannot engage in normal market behavior. They do not have sufficient information about the quality of physicians and hospitals to search for high quality relative to costs. Moreover, consumers are reluctant to change physicians because they develop personal relationships and because medical care is often given in emergency or stressful situations. As medical technology becomes steadily more complex and the rate of technological change accelerates, all these problems of consumer evaluation are exacerbated (see Figure 8.2).

There are two other imperfections in medical markets. The first is that good medical care is highly valued, and most individuals are disinclined to alter their purchases of medical care on the basis of price. Even when prices increase, patient behavior vis-à-vis providers changes little. The second is that if people do not have medical insurance, their ability to purchase health care is often severely limited, especially as medical costs continue to skyrocket. Since an estimated thirty-five million Americans presently do not have insurance, there is a serious problem of access. Despite appearances, these two imperfections are not contradictory. Even though most everyone wants good medical care, and a high proportion will pay very high prices for it, it is also

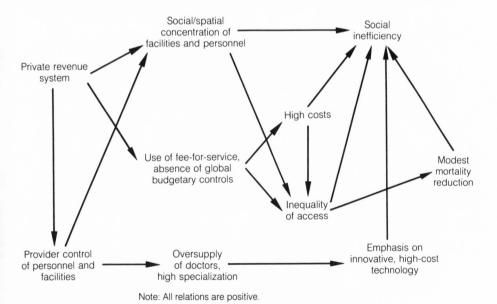

Note: All relations are positive.

Figure 8.2. The Logic of Privatization in Medical Care

true that many who do not qualify for Medicaid or Medicare in the United States do not have the means to pay for the medical care they need. The consequence is impoverishment and lower levels of health for many citizens, with many implications for policies. Before we address this issue, we also want to explore the logic of state intervention.

State managers, operating with substantial (albeit variable) autonomy, pursue a mix of policy goals with a different logic, sometimes supporting the preferences of providers, sometimes of consumers. This logic is best understood by examining the consequences of some of the mechanisms by which the state exerts control (see Figure 8.3).

State control over the appointment of personnel increases the probability that the regional distribution of medical personnel will be better balanced than it is in a privatized system. Because physicians are highly trained and enjoy high status, they tend to prefer urban contexts, leading to serious regional imbalances in the distribution of medical resources in privatized systems. This kind of institutional failure increases the likelihood that states will intervene to ensure that physicians and other resources are more equitably distributed. State control over both prices and personnel also tends to make medical care more widely affordable and accessible. In the chapter on equality, we observed how increased state funding of medical care in Great Britain and the United States led to the creation of such programs as National Health Insurance, the National Health Service, Medicaid, and Medicare and how

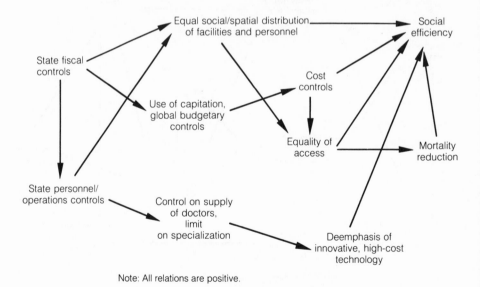

Note: All relations are positive.

Figure 8.3. The Logic of State Intervention in Medical Care

these programs resulted in higher numbers of patient visits to physicians and admissions to hospitals, especially for the poor and the elderly.

State control over prices, personnel, and revenues increases the availability of medical services and thus explains how state intervention reduces mortality. We are aware that this argument is somewhat contrary to that of McKeown and others, who contend that medical technology and other forms of medical intervention have had very modest effects in lowering mortality rates during the past century, that the decline in mortality was due to a rise in the standard of living, primarily improved diet. Nevertheless, these changes were mediated by changes in medical knowledge and state intervention, without which improvements in diet and other standard-of-living indicators might have had very modest effects.

State intervention has substantial effects on medical costs as well. If the state simply provides the revenue for medical services without attempting to regulate how the revenues are used, the demand for medical services soars and medical expenditures rise markedly. Historically, states have turned to financing first, and efforts to regulate prices and personnel, because of the power of medical providers, have been more modest. Once the state begins to provide revenues, and bureaucrats acquire knowledge about the delivery of medical services, they tend to become more involved in regulating prices and personnel. This pattern is consistent with the findings of recent literature inspired by Hugh Heclo and Theda Skocpol, which demonstrates that social policy is incrementally shaped by state bureaucrats and reformist intellectuals who learn from their previous experience (Heclo, 1974; Skocpol and Amenta, 1986; Skocpol and Ikenberry, 1983; Amenta et al., 1984; Evans et al., 1985; Orloff, 1985; Orloff and Skocpol, 1984). In short, the greater the state's involvement in funding, the greater its control over prices and personnel and the more effective its ability to limit the rise in medical spending.

State control can reduce prices in several ways. The state can plan the location of different kinds of hospitals on the basis of their ability to handle common to rare forms of illnesses and accidents, for example, reducing the duplication common to market systems, in which hospitals compete for physicians and indirectly for patients. This single factor helps explain much of the higher per capita medical costs in the United States compared to Great Britain. Furthermore, the state can regulate expenditures on medical consumption not only by rationing capital equipment but by regulating the number of physicians who can receive degrees and the proportion who can become specialists. One of the reasons why Sweden spends more per capita than Great Britain on medical care is that Sweden has exercised less control over specialization.

Contrary to those scholars who maintain that the marketplace is the most efficient institutional arrangement for the delivery of medical services, we found that privatization leads to higher spending for medical services without compensating improvement in levels of health. Privatized systems generate too many imbalances in the distribution of physicians, plants, and equipment, and in the consumption of medical services. State intervention mitigates these failures, though rationing of services also leads to greater bureaucratization, standardization, and waiting time.

Human Capital and Complex Technology

State intervention alone does not determine the performance of medical delivery systems, nor is state intervention the sole prescription for current dilemmas. Investments in human capital and technological complexity have also had dramatic effects on performance, and these lie at the core of many contemporary policy debates. What is unusual about our analysis is that we have attempted to control for human capital and social development in evaluating the effectiveness and efficiency of state intervention.

Scholars continue to debate the efficacy of investment in human capital. At a theoretical level, Ivar Berg (1970), Randall Collins (1979), and other have found that investment in human capital leads to status inflation through credentialing, with little or no payoff for improved system performance. Their general hypothesis applies to medical care as well. Between 1890 and 1970 medical knowledge has become embodied in an elaborate system of human capital (including medical research and specialization) and increasingly capital-intensive and expensive technology. But have increases in the number of doctors and the proportion of specialists improved levels of health or the social efficiency of medical systems, or have they been socially inefficient and inflationary influences?

In some nations the state has actively regulated and restricted the trend toward specialization and "high-technology" care generated by the very rapidly increasing body of medical knowledge. In other nations, particularly the United States, neither state policy nor private-sector regulation such as board certification has been able to arrest these tendencies. The American medical establishment, recognizing that medical specialization and technology have gotten out of control, is beginning to struggle with how the "oversupply" of subspecialists might be controlled (Petersdorf, 1985; Schwartz et al., 1988).

In each of the four countries, the number of medical personnel and medical treatment facilities has expanded substantially from 1890 to the present. More important, the knowledge base and technological complexity of "scientific medicine" have undergone striking changes during this time, especially since World War II. Knowledge of diseases and disease vectors has increased, and treatments believed to be highly efficacious exist for many of the conditions that were major contributors to morbidity and mortality in 1890. This expansion of knowledge has contributed to the dominance of "scientific" medicine over other models and to the steady increase in the differentiation and specialization of medical personnel and treatment facilities. Such changes, as we have demonstrated, have had considerable consequences for the performance of medical delivery systems, both in conjunction with larger societal changes and independently of them.

Evaluating the social costs and benefits of state intervention compared to privatized forms of coordination, we found striking differences, depending upon the type of state intervention. State control over revenues and state control over prices and personnel, although interrelated, do not have the same consequences. In contrast, the number of physicians per 100,000 population and the proportion of specialists affect medical performance the same way (see Table 8.2). Our findings suggest, contrary to the suggestions of the most radical critics (e.g., Illich, 1976), that physician supply and the complexity of medical technology do improve levels of health and directly reduce mortality rates. Since we have controlled for a wide variety of factors that also affect population mortality, most notably indicators of the standard of living, this result calls for some modification of McKeown's interpretation (1975, 1976). Many of the effects of a rising standard of living on levels of health are in fact mediated through physicians, who disseminate knowledge about diet, sanitation, and other public health measures. The quantity of physicians has had more effect in lowering mortality than McKeown and some others have previously estimated. Also, higher levels of medical education and advanced training lower mortality somewhat. Thus, there is some merit to the view that higher levels of specialization lead to higher levels of population health. On the other hand, a high level of medical specialization is often related to inequality of access. Under private systems, specialists and sophisticated technology tend toward geographical concentration and high consumer cost. Both tendencies may limit the access of lower-income consumers to the fruits of the technological advances.

The number of physicians and the proportion of specialists indirectly drive up medical costs because demand for medical care is partially self-generating. Since the general practitioner is the gatekeeper to

Table 8.2. Total Assessment of Investment in Human Capital

Performance	Number of physicians per 100,000 population			Proportion of specialists		
	Direct path coefficients	Net effects	Qualitative assessment	Direct path coefficients	Net effects	Qualitative assessment
Costs	+	+	+	+	+	+
Mortality	−	−	−	−	−	−
Social efficiency	−	−	−	−	−	−
Innovativeness Diffusion time of immunizations[a]	−	−	−	−	−	−

	Qualitative assessments	
	Number of physicians per 100,000 population	Proportion of specialists
Innovativeness Diffusion time of high-cost technologies	−	−
Equality Access to care	+	−
Regional equalization of services	+	−

[a]Based on data presented in Figure 5.2.

medical care, the larger the number of physicians, the greater the access to care and the more services a population receives. The number of visits to physicians per capita and, indeed, physician fees also rise as the number of physicians increases. Likewise, some have suggested that the more hospital beds there are, the more they are used. In short, supply generates its own demand in the medical area and tends to be relatively insensitive to price (Fuchs and Kramer, 1972; Evans, 1974; and for a critique of this position, see Sloan and Feldman, 1978; Enthoven, 1980). Increasing the number of physicians increases costs.

The net effect of increasing human capital investment and technological complexity has been to reduce social efficiency. The gains in lower mortality have been more than offset by rising costs, regardless of standards of living and variations in the form and extent of state coordination of medical services.

Human capital and technological complexity also affect system innovativeness, the speed of diffusion of both low-cost, highly efficacious technologies demanded by almost everyone and expensive technologies demanded by only a few. In both cases, controlling for other variables, increases in the number of physicians and in the proportion of specialists increased the speed of diffusion.

Physicians also shape system innovativeness through their power vis-à-vis the state. Physicians in every country constitute a strong interest group, able to limit state intervention or to influence the form it takes. Our analyses suggest that if physicians use their influence to block or limit state intervention, expensive technologies diffuse more rapidly, costs rise, and social efficiency declines. On the other hand, if the state succeeds in establishing control over the appointment of personnel and medical prices, the diffusion of expensive technologies and costs can be constrained, and thus social efficiency rises.

Despite the substantial and important contributions of growing medical knowledge and the developing medical system to population health, there have been a number of undesirable side effects. Overall, increases in human capital investment reduce social efficiency and may deprive many of access to services. There appears to be a point beyond which returns on investment in human capital and specialization are not socially efficient. These findings are consistent with the views of some that status inflation has occurred among doctors in the United States. A much higher proportion of American physicians are specialists than is the case in most European societies. We suggest that very limited state intervention and reliance on market mechanisms facilitate credentialing in the United States. State intervention, whether to limit or promote the growth of human capital, may be highly relevant to the policy problems arising from the development of medical technology. By slowing investment, credentialing may be restricted, resulting in greater returns to investment in human capital, reduced system costs, and enhanced social efficiency.

But reducing the number of physicians and the proportion of physicians who are specialists may have less favorable effects as well. If there were fewer doctors and specialists, most likely there would be a decline in the information about health and a corresponding decline in levels of health. On the other hand, if the state distributed physicians and specialists so that consumers had even better access to care, levels of health could improve, even with fewer doctors.

The diffusion of innovation would also be affected, for technologies would spread less rapidly, perhaps producing cost savings in the short term. Without state intervention, reductions in the numbers of physicians and specialists would also reduce access to medical services. Both spatial and class inequalities would rise. Without the state to guide the process, such reductions are likely to have socially unacceptable consequences. Again, it is not privatization but greater and more thoughtful state coordination that would probably extract more positive performance from medical delivery systems.

Social Development

We have stressed the importance of state intervention and the complexity of medical technology in defining the central crises that underlie contemporary policy debates, but it should not be forgotten that the performance of medical systems and the problems they confront are in very large part products of the societal environment in which they operate. Neither the performance problems nor the range of possible alternatives are the same as we approach 1990 as they were when we entered the era of "scientific medicine" in the 1890s. The intervening period witnessed unprecedented changes in the material prosperity of Western nations. Controlling for inflation, per capita income has doubled and redoubled in each of the four countries, making possible the allocation of large sums of money to medical care. Work was transformed from primarily agricultural labor performed by family units to industrial labor in large factories, and finally to employment in a vastly expanded service sector. As the nature of work, family, employment, and property relations were transformed, so were the medical needs and vulnerabilities of entire populations. And it was in response to these changes that organizational changes of medical systems occurred.

Another critical part of the evolving societal environment was the perceptions, desires, and understandings of the populations. Between 1890 and 1980, popular beliefs about health, curative medical care, and "scientific medicine" changed substantially, as did beliefs about how medical care ought to be organized. Mass public education, the increasing dominance of the "scientific" model, and the rationalization of culture through the increasing role exercised by large organizations in the structuring of everyday life have also played a large, if subtler role in the transformation of medical systems.

To complete our analysis, we show in Table 8.3 the direct and net effects of social development. Many of the influences of social development are indirect, mediated by other variables. On balance, social development has little independent effect on mortality. The aging of the population offsets the gains of rising levels of income and education and their impact on health consciousness and styles of life. While social development is at the root of long-term reduction in population mortality, some of its effects cancel out others, and most effects appear to be mediated by state intervention and medical system development. So-

Table 8.3. Total Assessment of Investment of
Social Development

Performance	Direct path coefficients	Net effects
Costs	+	+
Mortality	Nil*	−
Social efficiency	−	−

*Nil effect is defined as < .05.

cial development does, however, lead to more spending on medical care. As many have said, the steady rise in the standard of living has permitted a shift in the proportion of money allocated to medical care. Similarly, net of the impact of investment in human capital and of both state intervention variables, social development has reduced the diffusion time of new medical advances.

Taking all these connections into account, we conclude that social development has had a moderately negative effect on the social efficiency of medical systems because it has little direct effect on mortality but a moderately positive effect on costs. Nevertheless, the long-term decline in social efficiency is less than one might expect. The negative effects of social development on the social efficiency of medical systems have been partly limited by more effective state intervention, which is itself partially a consequence of social development. Increasing wealth and education, along with many other factors, have increased the capacity of lower-income consumers to demand greater access to medical services. The increased state intervention that has historically developed from efforts to broaden access has also given state managers some leverage over the operation of medical systems, often resulting in greater social efficiency.

Policy Implications

What are the policy implications of this research? We propose to confront this question first by discussing the kind of system which seems inadvisable. We will then suggest various strategies that are likely to maximize system performance, although with the caveat that existing structural arrangements in each society and the relative power of groups may make certain policy alternatives impossible. Moreover, it is difficult to maximize all performances simultaneously, for some are incompatible. For example, a highly efficient system is not likely to be very innovative, and a system that has achieved an egalitarian distribution of standardized general services is not likely to be highly flexible and adaptive to costly new technologies. There are tradeoffs among system performances, and each society must select those it considers most important, maximizing as many as possible.

Privatized systems are less rigid than state-managed systems, and they tend to provide a higher quality of care for upper-income groups, but despite their common image of efficiency, they are, in fact, socially inefficient. Privatized systems, particularly market-oriented ones, are characterized by geographical maldistribution of resources; they are inegalitarian and prone to cost inflation and priority distortion; they generate lower levels of health in the aggregate and an emphasis on curative as opposed to preventive forms of medicine (Rodwin, 1984; Alford, 1975; Hollingsworth, 1986; Abel-Smith, 1976; Weller and Manga, 1983). This is not to say that there is no room for private-sector organizations, even in statist systems. Indeed, the flexibility of private organizations means that all societies benefit by having some medical services in the private sector.

Despite the evidence demonstrating the inadequate performance of national medical systems organized predominantly in the private sector, there are advocates of privatization on both sides of the Atlantic. Somewhat ironically, this view has most adherents in the United States, where the consequences of privatization are most prominent. Of the four countries examined herein, the United States most fully realizes the performance tendencies of privatized medicine, and it is, therefore, the least socially efficient and egalitarian.

In the United States, there is considerable competition for patients among different types of private providers (HMOs, hospitals, etc.). New knowledge and technology, for example, now permit many procedures that formerly were done in the hospital to be done in the office of the physician. In parts of the United States, the competition between hospitals and physicians in outpatient clinics has become quite intense. The average cost of those procedures that can be performed on an ambulatory basis has indeed declined, but the incidence of such procedures has increased dramatically, and as many new technologies have stabilized, the costs have begun to rise. Some estimate that almost half of all surgical procedures are performed on an outpatient basis. Despite the undoubted savings on hospital costs per procedure, competition between doctor-owned clinics and hospitals has led to no overall savings. Moreover, ambulatory services that occur in the privacy of a physician's office without the scrutiny of peer review and with the assistance of those employed directly by the surgeon raise critical questions about the quality of care (Goldsmith, 1981; Reinhardt, 1975; Davis and Detmar, 1972).

For some years, many have advocated a privatized, highly competitive structure of health maintenance organizations as a means of reducing medical costs. Research is demonstrating, however, that HMOs compete with one another on the basis of amenities and conveniences at the expense of efficiency (Abel-Smith, 1985). Again we see the perversities of market tendencies in the medical area. Rather than promote optimal levels of care at reasonable prices, the competitive HMO institutional arrangement has thus far resulted in too much care at too much cost with unnecessary duplication and dubious efficiency and quality.

It has become increasingly apparent that the strategy of increasing competition and privatization has not been accomplishing its goals in the United States. Many medical professionals and policy makers now express concern about the large numbers of Americans who have been left out of the system of private insurance; raise questions about the quality of care provided to those who do have insurance; and complain that physicians are losing autonomy and control as private-sector "regulation" by hospital corporations, HMO management, and insurance firms is added to state regulation (Kinzer, 1988).

Nor has "competition" restrained the growth of medical costs. At the beginning of 1988 the Health Insurance Association of America reported that premiums for those Americans fortunate enough to have medical insurance would rise by 10 to 70 percent, and the main governmental insurance program (Medicare) raised its premiums by nearly 40 percent (*New York Times*, January 12, 1988; McCarthy, 1988). Contrary to the expectations of "privatizers," the reforms to create greater competitiveness in the American system have driven prices up, not down. The American case may be an extreme example of the contradictions and failures of privatization because of the high degree of specialization in the system and the weak, limited, and uncoordinated historical role of the state. Nevertheless, the tragic failure of the system eloquently illustrates our conclusion that reliance on private-oriented mechanisms to coordinate the production and delivery of medical services limits access to care and produces redundancy and inefficiency in the system while driving up costs.

It is true, of course, that Americans could modify the system without abandoning privatization, but the reader should be aware that such efforts during the past decade have not prevented the system from becoming more costly, less socially efficient, and less egalitarian. Perhaps some specific characteristics of the American system will help to dramatize its poor performance.[1]

1. In preparing this discussion of the recent performance of the American medical system, we are indebted to Joel Rogers, "Caring for America: A Progressive Health Care Policy Agenda" (unpublished paper, Madison, Wisconsin). Also see Hollingsworth and

By 1988, the United States was spending 11 percent of its gross national product on medical care, but as the costs have increased, the proportion of Americans who lack the means to purchase adequate care has also increased. Historically, those who could not pay were subsidized by higher charges to those who could pay. In recent years, however, government and large employers, in order to reduce their costs, have been refusing to participate in cross-subsidization. As a result, hospitals that historically served the poor are now being fiscally squeezed. Many are having to close; others are cutting back on unprofitable services. Meantime, government budgets, in response to the fiscal crisis of the state, are either reducing indigent care or are failing to respond to public needs. The overall result is a serious lack of access for low-income Americans.

Approximately 35 million Americans presently have no medical insurance—almost one of every six Americans under age sixty-five. Another 20 million have such inadequate insurance that a major illness would lead to bankruptcy. Indeed, almost 17 million Americans who are gainfully employed lack health insurance—up from 14 million in 1982. Each year, approximately 1 million people are denied medical care for financial reasons, and approximately 200,000 are turned away from hospital emergency rooms. Annually, half a million mothers have no form of medical insurance when they give birth, 1.3 million pregnant women get insufficient prenatal care, and 11 million children are not covered by any form of medical insurance. Nor do children receive the school health inspections that the British began more than seventy years ago. Older Americans are the only group covered by comprehensive public health insurance, but they now pay as large a share of their income on medical care as they did before Medicare was implemented in 1965.

There are many other indications that medical care is becoming less accessible. Since 1980, the number of Americans without medical insurance has increased by 7 million people. Only 45 percent of the poor are covered by Medicaid, in contrast to 65 percent in 1976. During the past ten years, the infant mortality rate has increased in more than a dozen states. As the squeeze to control prices has increased, copayments and deductibles have risen, with the average person now paying 27 percent of health care costs. Moreover, many who are insured cannot plan on remaining insured. For example, 75 percent of workers over age forty-five who lost their jobs during the 1982 recession lost their medical insurance as well. In the past, unionized workers in manufacturing jobs

Hollingsworth 1987; and *New York Times*, June 23, 1988, August 21, 1988, September 9, 1988.

had the best coverage among people in the work force, but as the economy has shifted from manufacturing to service and the level of unionization has declined, the proportion of the population with adequate medical insurance has also gone down. Those with preexisting diseases frequently cannot obtain medical insurance without paying astronomical rates.

In sum, the peculiar mix of privatization and state intervention in the United States is leading to unparalleled spending and inadequate access to care. No country in the world now spends a higher proportion of its gross national product on medical care than does the United States. Yet in no other industrial country are so many denied medical services, and there is mounting evidence that the health of low-income Americans is declining. For the past sixty years health planners have portrayed the system as being in a crisis. Certainly, in 1990 the system appears to be closer to a crisis than it has ever been (Alford, 1975).

If societies are to give all or nearly all citizens access to care, improve health care in the aggregate, limit increases in medical costs, and increase the efficiency of their medical delivery systems, the state must play a major role in both historical forms of intervention: regulating activity on the demand side and controlling the supply of services. These approaches, as we have demonstrated, have markedly different consequences for system performance.

Most countries have tried to restrain the demand for medical care by requiring individuals to pay for some services. In the United States, this payment is usually labeled copayment, deductibles, or coinsurance. In other countries it is often called cost sharing or charges on the customers. In some countries this kind of policy has applied primarily to drugs and eye glasses; in others it has applied to almost all services. Unfortunately, such "demand side" manipulations, which operate to the particular disadvantage of the poor, the aged, and the chronically ill, have proven rather ineffective in restraining cost growth. In general, organizational efforts to decrease demand have not been very successful.

By contrast, state regulation on the supply side has been more successful in enhancing the cost-effectiveness of medical delivery systems through a variety of strategies. Some governments have attempted to limit the supply of physicians, hospitals, and other facilities and to control resource allocation (Abel-Smith, 1976:154–60). Governments have also attempted to control supply by specifying the prices that will be paid for specific services. Some governments have required prior approval before certain services are provided. Other have established programs to guarantee that medical services are necessary and of high quality in order for reimbursement to take place.

Although supply manipulations have generally proven more effective than those on the demand side in the contemporary period, one of the major weaknesses in government policy in various countries has been haphazard planning and poor linkage between those who plan for the delivery of services and those who pay for services. For example, in the United States the Health Care Financing Administration has coordinated the financing of Medicare programs but has had very little to do with shaping the supply of physicians, hospitals, and other facilities. This, like other American regulatory bodies, has been superimposed on existing structures rather than integrated into a single system.

The failure to coordinate supply with demand manipulations may, in fact, have further distorted the priorities of the American system beyond the failures generated by the market. Because the relative power of providers has not changed substantially even though the American state has funded care of the elderly and indigent, the system has fostered the performances preferred by providers (see Figure 8.1). In Great Britain, by contrast, the state has effectively linked supply planning and financing by integrating the entire system. The lower degree of unified control in the French and Swedish systems may be a factor in their higher costs and lower levels of social efficiency. Swedish hospitals are organized at the county level, but manpower controls are exercised by the central government, for example. Hence, the county may expand a hospital but depends on the national government for the approval of medical staff to work in the hospital. Even so, the various county councils finance almost half of Sweden's medical expenditures, reflecting weak central control and coordination. To promote greater efficiency, the national government has superimposed regional planning on the counties, but many traditional decentralized structures have persisted, and the Swedes have had great difficulty in controlling medical expenditures (Rodwin, 1984:56–57, 236–37).

To be equitable and efficient, a system requires state control over not just one but all of the following: the financing of medical care, the distribution of resources, and the supply of manpower. There are several strategies that the state might employ to achieve these ends. First, primarily to control costs, the state might eliminate reimbursement on a fee-for-service basis and develop salary or capitation reimbursement, thus reducing incentives to prescribe costly medical services. Tendencies in this direction can be observed in the medical systems of each of the highly developed countries. Second, governments might end free entry by doctors to specialization to prevent serious misallocations in the distribution of the doctors across specialties, which leads to unnecessary surgery and other forms of treatment. Many countries now restrict both the number of medical school graduates and the number who may specialize in particular fields. Third, governments might provide financial incentives to encourage doctors to locate in rural areas. Similarly, in "overdoctored" areas, the state, as a financier of physicians services, may pay doctors lower fees for services or make lower capitation payments. Great Britain has long had a system of negative controls, whereby general practitioners have not been permitted to locate in areas designated as overdoctored. Controls have not completely solved the problem of geographical maldistribution of practitioners, but they have mitigated it (Davis, 1977; Rodwin, 1984; Abel-Smith, 1976).

Advocates of privatization suggest that state intervention in medical care has been relatively ineffective and has often failed to accomplish its intended results, and we are inclined to agree. In most of the Western nations, particularly the United States, state intervention has tended to occur in response to problems (rather than to prevent them), has sought to manipulate system performance primarily through financial incentives (rather than by direct regulation), and has mainly focused on the demand side of medical exchanges, rather than also manipulating the supply.

Nevertheless, deregulation or privatization of medical systems will not remedy the failures and limitations of the current systems of state intervention. The more promising strategy is to make state intervention more effective. In particular, the state must focus more attention on such supply considerations as the quantity, quality, and location of medical production. Effective mechanisms must be created to integrate and coordinate manipulations of the supply with such demand manipulations as entitlements, pricing, etc. And the state must use its regulatory and legal power to accomplish policy objectives, rather than rely on the public purse for market incentives to providers and consumers.

These proposals may appear radical to Americans but quite mild to Europeans. They address only a part of the problem of how to provide for greater societal health in the contemporary period, however. Many of the more fundamental difficulties cannot be met through simple adjustments (however radical) to the current structure of delivering medical services. For continued improvement of societal health, it will be increasingly necessary to transform the structure and goals of medical delivery systems while supporting and curing those who are ill.

Efficiency and equality are likely to be served by limits on the power the state had earlier granted to medical professionals, which would move systems away from physician-dominated, expensive medical high technology toward manpower substitution, comprehensive health centers, salary and capitation payment of medical providers, limited diffusion of expensive technology, and utilization-review committees. If the state begins to use its resources to develop balanced and comprehensive institutions in a single site, it will be possible for the elderly and mental patients to receive better medical care when they need it. Balanced medical centers would help to guarantee that researchers, teachers, clinicians, and students would have contact with a much broader range of illness and populations and not just the narrow range of cases that researchers and teachers have historically viewed as interesting. It is important that there be sufficient restructuring of medical education and treatment centers so that medical personnel will be sensitive to the full range of problems influencing health. There might then be increasing realization that medical education requires more of a partnership between the medical profession and other professions (for example, engineers, architects, city planners, social workers, state officials, and lawyers), united to prevent and cope with disease.

This restructuring is not likely to occur through a privatized system. Only the state has the authority to bring it about. With such change, there is potential that the systems will behave differently on the various performance indicators. Given the distribution of power among groups in each country, however, it remains to be seen whether the state has the capacity to bring about this kind of structural change and hence to alter system performance substantially. Variation among countries in the historical distribution of power among key groups guarantees that even if all four states confront these problems, they will attempt to solve them in very different ways.

The Changing American Environment

At the beginning of this chapter, we suggested that the relative power of particular interest groups and the coalitions they form help to explain why particular arrangements exist in a society. Currently, in the United States a power shift is under way which increases the probability of more state intervention despite the various pleas for privatization. In contrast to the medical systems in the other countries, the American case is striking for the lack of state coordination among various parts of the system, the considerable regional variation in system characteristics and performance, and the lack of policy "coherence" among functional areas of decision making. For example, decisions about personnel, access, and supply of equipment are less well coordinated with decisions about prices and costs of care than in the other three countries. Because of the lack of coherence, comprehensive administrative authority, and ideological consensus, the Americans attempt to accomplish a great deal through monetary incentives, rather than direct command. This approach has proven remarkably unsuccessful in controlling costs, equalizing access, and achieving social efficiency.

There are those who argue that if incentives were properly established in the private sector, different kinds of performances would follow. Given the existing structure of the American system, however, a fundamentally different set of incentives is not likely to emerge. Thus, the Americans eagerly and continuously pass legislation in hopes of establishing new incentives and of improving system performance, but of course, disappointments persist as the legislation fails to achieve stated goals. Americans are not likely to be successful unless the underlying structure of the system is altered. In the final analysis, it is institutional change that is likely to have the greatest impact in modifying system performance. The difficult task is to transform the ways that low- and upper-income consumers, providers, employers, insurers, and regulators view societal health and the role of medical care. Only through overhaul of the institutional arrangement and goals of the medical system can Americans hope to continue to improve health into the twenty-first century.

As Americans ponder the rather poor performance of their medical system, they probably have more capacity to bring about a fundamental restructuring than at any time during the past seventy years. According to one of the central insights of institutional analysts, institutional arrangements are very much shaped by their social environment. The key environmental factor is the relative power of the main actors, which has changed profoundly in the United States.

Since 1965, governmental bureaucrats—especially those paying the bills of Medicare—have become extraordinarily knowledgeable about the costs of care throughout the nation. Inasmuch as those who pay the bills eventually wish to regulate prices as well as the actual delivery of services, we can now expect the American state to become much more interventionist. Even the Reagan presidency—which advocated deregulation and a weak state—introduced the diagnostic related grouping system and thus did more than any administration in American history to intervene in the actual practice of medicine. Meantime, employers such as General Motors, Ford, and other large corporations are using their buying power with insurance carriers to develop alternative methods of organizing and financing medical care in the United States. As the costs of medical insurance have assumed an even larger share of funds that might otherwise be available for wage increases, large labor unions are increasingly using their leverage to develop alternative means of financing, organizing, and promoting better health. Finally, whereas seventy years ago, the American Medical Association was the dominant actor in the delivery of health care, its power to shape medical policy has greatly diminished as the state, big capital, and organized labor have developed a vested interest in controlling costs and promoting a more socially efficient medical system. In the financial squeeze, hospitals adopt an agenda that significantly diverges from that of doctors. Moreover, doctors are far more differentiated than they were sixty years ago—fragmented not only into specialties but also split between private practitioners and those employed by various corporate entities (HMOs, large clinics, universities, etc.). Although doctors may still be the most powerful group in shaping American medical policy, they have much less clout than formerly, and this restructuring of power within the environment of the American medical system will ultimately lead to new institutional arrangements for the delivery of medical care.

The direction change will take in American society is at present uncertain, but we end this book with a certain degree of optimism. Crises generate the potential for new institutional arrangements. The process of educating the citizenry about better health is already under way. How medical problems are defined, however, and the strategies for solving them will be shaped by all the actors: providers, consumers, and the state.

Observations about the European Medical Systems

Recent data on medical expenditures as a percentage of gross national product reveal that the three European countries retain rankings similar to those of 1970. Britain has the lowest expenditures, with France next, and Sweden and the United States the most.

The performance of these systems has implications for policy considerations. France and Sweden have relatively strong states, capable of more effective coordination of their medical systems, but both countries have had inadequate state coordination and control of their hospital systems. The French have considerable excess capacity in hospital beds, almost twice as many hospital beds per 100,000 people as the United States, but a much lower admission rate. By most indicators, the French have a socially inefficient hospital system, lacking coordination between demand for hospital beds and supply.

Sweden also has excess supply in its medical sector. At present, it has almost 2.5 times as many hospital beds per capita as the United States and approximately 70 percent more doctors per capita than Britain. Among the four countries, the Swedes admit the highest proportion of the population to hospitals and have the longest average length of stay (Organization for Economic Cooperation and Development, 1985).

But overall, the Swedish system performs quite well relative to the other three countries. It is clearly the most egalitarian of the four systems. The Swedish population has easy access to low-cost standardized services demanded by many, and those needing high-cost technologies have easy access to them. Moreover, the latest technologies tend to diffuse throughout Sweden very rapidly. Most observers consider the quality of Swedish ambulatory and hospital services to be exceptionally high.

Relative to other countries, the weakness of the Swedish system is the high level of expenditure (approximately 11 percent of gross national product) on medical care. In part, high spending is a reflection of poor coordination by the Swedish state. A substantial portion of the Swedish medical system is financed by county councils. With both the national government and local agencies responsible for medical provision, there are many points at which pressures are exerted to increase expenditures. Because medical care is the most significant responsibility of the county councils—comprising a small number of politicians who determine expenditure levels and countywide priorities—medical decisions have high local visibility and invite a great deal of public discussion. A high degree of local autonomy among county councils has done much to promote equality of access and excellence in the quality of care. If the Swedes wish to reduce their level of expenditures, however, our study suggests that movement toward privatization is not the answer, even though many Swedish doctors are calling for greater privatization in an effort to enhance their autonomy and income. The most effective means of constraining rising costs would be greater control over the entire system by the central government, probably feasible in the relatively small Swedish system. Such control would probably reduce duplication, as well as the speed of diffusion of costly new technologies. Under more centralized control, upper-income groups would probably have less influence on the governance of the system, slightly reducing its legitimacy. On the other hand, the power of the Social Democratic party and lower-income groups would probably be enhanced.

Although Britain has the most socially efficient system, there is considerable dissatisfaction among upper-income groups and doctors. One major source of this dissaffection is the stringent constraint on expenditures, which results in modest incomes for doctors, long waiting time for elective surgery, and an inadequate supply of doctors, specialists, hospital beds, and many high-cost technologies. In our judgment, fiscal constraints are excessive, and more resources need to be expended. The situation in Britain underscores an important point: a national medical system may be socially efficient and quite egalitarian, but it can also generate a great deal of inconvenience at the individual level—more, indeed, than is necessary. Confronted with the interesting problem of what the appropriate level of medical expenditure is, relative to a specific age-sex population pyramid and the level of economic development, the British—at approximately 6 percent of GNP—are probably spending too little, whereas the United States and Sweden—at over 10 percent—may be spending too much. Regardless of the answer, it is useful to ponder with cross-national data the question of the proper balance between the social efficiency of the total system and the convenience for individuals.

Not only would the British system benefit by allocating more resources for medical care, but the legitimacy and the overall quality of the system could be enhanced if greater flexibility were introduced. One of the major problems confronting consumers of medical care is inadequate knowledge about the performance of specific parts of their system. The American government has demonstrated that it is possible to develop profiles about the services delivered by different types of providers—hospitals, doctors, etc. Since most of the British system is financed by the state, the government could also develop profiles on the quality of services and the waiting times for them. The more the state is involved in the coordination and control of medical care, the greater its capacity to collect information about the quality of specific types of services and to share it with consumers. As a result of this information, general practitioners and patients could make better-informed decisions about the availability and quality of specialized treatments. Moreover, hospitals with inadequate resources or services could more easily be singled out for public scrutiny. Because hospitals should thereafter be funded on the basis of their performance, this process could introduce incentives and competition into a state system. There would be market-type activity in the National Health Service without the necessity of moving to privatization, which would probably lead to greater inequalities in access. While this kind of sharing of information may invite constant public pressures for reform, the dissemination of this kind of information seems most appropriate in a democratic society—especially in an economic sector in which consumers have great difficulty in making informed decisions about where to seek treatment.

One of the most interesting aspects of modern medical care is its institutional failure in the general area of social equality. Although all four systems have over time provided greater equality of access to medical care, efforts to reduce inequality in levels of health across social classes and income groups have been much less successful. Our study suggests that states cannot have much impact on equalizing levels of health across social classes and income groups unless they invest heavily in public health education, especially in programs targeted for the working class. In such preventive measures as discouraging smoking and poor dietary habits, banning leaded gas, and controlling use of nonleaded gas, pollution in urban areas, the British and the French have lagged far behind the Swedish and American governments in trying to modify destructive behaviors. Sweden remains a model in this area, probably because the beginnings of the Swedish medical system were in the public sector.

France has been especially reluctant to regulate destructive life styles. For example, automobile fatalities for every 100,000 miles driven are much higher in France than in the other three countries. French morbidity and death due to cirrhosis of the liver are also much higher. Because Britain and France have substantial state involvement in the delivery of medical care, they have considerable potential for educating the working class via family physicians and various social agencies. In general, preventive medicine has remained a major weakness of the British, French, and American systems because these societies have failed to eliminate widespread poverty and major inequalities in levels of education. Health education and preventive care deserve much higher emphasis than they have hitherto received.

Finally, we have an observation for future research on national medical systems. This book has emphasized the role of human capital and state intervention in shaping levels of social efficiency. Each of the four systems, however, has inefficiencies. Although the British system may be the most socially efficient, this certainly does not mean that it is the most efficient in each segment of its medical system. One useful area of future research is to explore particular kinds of inefficiencies and then attempt to reduce them. Because national medical systems vary in the way that they are inefficient, they should learn from each other.

State Intervention and Human Capital Paradigms

Throughout this book we have explicated two perspectives for analyzing social services: state intervention and human capital. We believe that these perspectives must be combined in any future social cost-benefit analysis at the level of the nation-state if there is to be an effective understanding of why particular institutional arrangements are likely to produce certain results. Evaluating institutional arrangements without considering the contribution of human capital, both quantity and quality, would lead to an overestimation of the contribution of the arrangement being considered. Simarily, looking at human capital without considering the nature of the institutional arrangements overlooks important insights.

Throughout this study, we have preferred to use the term *privatization* rather than markets, for the medical systems in these four countries have historically deviated from the neoclassical model of markets. The state has long licensed the practice of physicians and the behavior of hospitals. This form of state regulation is not part of our measure of state intervention because it is relatively constant across the four countries. Licensing, however, does reflect fundamental constraints on marketlike behavior. For these reasons, the term *privatization*—rather than markets—is a more appropriate concept for describing the institutional arrangements in the private sector of these countries. Of course, many advocates of privatization have assumed that the medical sector can operate as markets do in many other sectors of the economy, but we have demonstrated how the logic of privatization does not work as many of its advocates believe. And our section on the logic of privatization is an effort to advance the development of theory about institutional arrangements.

Our perspective on state intervention has four distinct components that can enrich the analysis not only of medical care but also of such other social services as education, mental health, welfare, and so forth. The first element is in conceptualizing the institutional arrangement called state intervention, an important problem in its own right. The theory of markets is well developed in the scholarly literature, but the theory of state hierarchies, as distinct from private hierarchies, needs much more work (Williamson, 1975, 1985; Lindblom, 1977). In the future we would like to examine more carefully the role of state bureaucrats in controlling prices and appointing personnel as well as in the financing of social services. Because we believe that state intervention at the local level, as in Sweden, is likely to have quite different consequences from intervention at the nation-state level, as in Britain, we see centralization as another area that needs more research and where our theoretical arguments can be pushed farther than we have done, though some scholarship exists on the subject (Hollingsworth and Hanneman, 1984).

A second component in our perspective is the specification of a wide range of performances and consideration of a social definition of an economic concept such as efficiency. The idea of social efficiency can be applied to many other kinds of social services, such as national standardized test scores in education or recidivism rates of prisons, juvenile delinquent homes, or mental hospitals. Such a perspective would allow scholars to perform social cost-benefit analysis without assigning some monetary value to particular social outcomes. Furthermore, our concept of social effectiveness has the same advantages and flexibility. It can be used in a wide variety of situations where profits or other economic measures are absent. Our analysis of social equality indicates how complex these performances can be. Institutional arrangements that provide equal access and regional equality do not necessarily provide equality of results. Perhaps in future research, it will be possible to incorporate other performance measures at the level of the nation-state.

A third element in our perspective is the specification of the logics of privatization and state intervention. In our analysis, we have stressed the processes of coordination and control, the relative power of particular groups, and the values of specific interest groups. As we demonstrated in our analysis of costs, privatization distributes power to particular actors, especially providers or professionals. Again, this insight has broad application for all kinds of social services, from education to mental health. Our analysis suggests that the power of psychiatrists, welfare workers, teachers, and so forth is much greater under some form of privatization. Even local government control allows less power to providers than a privatized system, limiting their ability to shape services and dictate costs. For example, our perspective offers suggestions as to why the costs of higher education are spiraling upward in the United States. The same variation in institutional arrangements which exists in the medical sector also exists in higher education and with the same consequences for social effectiveness, and social efficiency, and innovativeness. Much more work needs to be done on the logics of these institutional arrangements for other sectors. We believe, however, that we have begun to sketch the mechanisms the state uses to coordinate and control. This framework helps explain why different institutional arrangements lead to different performances.

The fourth component involves the values of particular interest groups relative to their preferences. Providers or professionals are not very interested in controlling costs. They like new technologies, even expensive ones, and are quite concerned about the quality of the service they provide. In contrast, state bureaucrats, who worry about the entire system, are likely to emphasize standardization and cost limits, especially since they also appreciate the political costs of government spending. Thus, they are persuaded by their own logic to control prices and the personnel, including the number of professionals. Finally, in sectors involving complex, rapidly changing technologies, consumers are not in a position to evaluate quality of service or to determine a fair price. As a consequence, they are generally powerless to influence performance except insofar as they can mobilize to bring about greater state intervention. This component completes the state intervention perspective by allowing one to ask why certain kinds of institutional arrangements prevail at particular historical moments in specific countries.

Together, these four components permit a more dynamic analysis of how crises produce new coalitions that then lead to new institutional arrangements, specifically state intervention (see Hollingsworth, 1986). We believe this general framework can incorporate a broader institutional analysis in various social science disciplines, though our main concern has been with developing a perspective for better understanding the delivery of social services, not all parts of an economy.

Scholars long ago demonstrated that the state intervenes in response to market failures. When it does, the relative power of particular groups almost always changes. Yet though we have been concerned with analyzing the consequences of state intervention, we realize that state intervention also has various drawbacks. Excessive state regulation can lead to rigid standardization and bureaucratization, possibly to a system that spends too little and is not very innovative—as with the British medical system. Again, we need more research: What are the upper limits to the advantages of state intervention? When do its attempts to coordinate become counterproductive?

Our framework is useful for evaluation of specific proposals for reform and to indicate whether they are likely to succeed and why. We have already provided an example of this kind of analysis in our consideration of the various proposals for privatization in medical care. This same framework can be employed in other sectors, but again, it is important to recognize that it must be at the level of the nation-state. Thus, one would focus on such performance as social effectiveness, social efficiency, and social equality of education, mental health, welfare services, child care, etc.

The interaction of the human capital and state intervention perspectives occurs at many points. To invest in some group of professionals does not just provide society with human capital but also creates a powerful interest group that fights to maintain its privileges. Its concerns about quality and technology and its lack of concerns about costs put upward pressure on the budget of the society. Institutional arrangements can give more or less power to state bureaucrats, consumers, and providers. Each of these interest groups desires different social benefits and is willing to accept different costs (Hollingsworth, 1986). Finally, the outcomes are a function not only of institutional arrangements but also of expertise. Therefore, the two paradigms need to be combined to reveal how social development occurs across time.

We believe we have a useful paradigm that allows institutional and policy analysis to consider the relative merits of state intervention in various social services. We also believe our perspective is as useful for policy makers as it is for academics interested in how to improve social services.

Appendix 1

SOURCES FOR TABLES[1]

Abbreviations Used in Source Citations

HSUS	*Historical Statistics of the United States,* parts 1 and 2 (Bureau of the Census, U.S. Department of Commerce, 1975).
SA	*Statistisk Arsbok* (Sweden, annual editions).
ASF	*Annuaire statistique de la France* (annual editions).
EHS	B. R. Mitchell, *European Historical Statistics, 1750–1970* (London: Macmillan, 1975); 2d rev. ed., *European Historical Statistics, 1750–1975* (New York: Facts on File, 1981).
HMSO	His/Her Majesty's Stationer's Office (London, unless noted).
GPO	Government Printing Office, Washington, D.C.
HEW	United States Department of Health, Education, and Welfare
MOH	Great Britain, Ministry of Health
IN	Imprimière Nationale, Paris, France

Sources for Table 2.1

The sources for these data are listed under Table 2.4.

Sources for Table 2.2

The index of state control over prices by degree of centralization was constructed from data on sources of revenue, listed under Table 2.4, which were modified to reflect the actual locus of price setting. For

---

1. For details on extrapolation, interpolation, graphing, and estimates, as well as other data adjustments, contact the authors.

example, although federal funds pay for the Medicare program, decisions about how the funds are spent are generally made in the private sector. Therefore, the Medicare amount, which appeared at the federal level on the revenue variable, is in the private sector on the prices variable. The index of personnel control was constructed from the following:

UNITED STATES

Department of Commerce, *Benevolent Institutions, 1904* (GPO, 1905, 1910); *HSUS*; U.S. Civil Service Commission, *Official Register of the United States* (GPO, 1891); *Directory of the American Medical Association,* I (Chicago: AMA, 1906); *American Medical Directory* (Chicago: AMA, 1912, 1921); U.S. Public Health Service, *Report of the Committee on Municipal Health Department Practice: Public Health Bulletin No. 136*; Department of Commerce, *Hospitals and Dispensaries, 1923* (GPO, 1925); Committee on the Cost of Medical Care, *Medical Care for the American People: Final Report* (Chicago: University of Chicago Press, 1932); Allan Peebles, *A Survey of Statistical Data on Medical Facilities in the United States* (Washington, D.C.: Committee on the Cost of Health Care, 1931); I. S. Falk et al., *The Costs of Medical Care* (Chicago: University of Chicago Press, 1931); H. G. Weiskotten, "Tendencies in Medical Practice," *Journal of the Association of American Medical Colleges* 7 (March 1932); *Health Manpower Source Book, No. 9: Physicians, Dentists, and Professional Nurses* (GPO, 1952); U.S. Public Health Service, *Distribution of Health Services in the Structure of State Government* (Washington, D.C.: U.S. Public Health Service, 1943); Haven Emerson and Martha Luginbuhl, "1200 Local Public Health Departments in the United States," *American Journal of Public Health* 35 (September 1945); HEW, *Public Health Service Publication No. 263* (GPO, 1959, 1961); *Journal of the American Hospital Association* 45, pt. 2 (August 1, 1971); William H. Stewart and Marion E. Attenderfer, *Health Manpower Source Book No. 13: Hospital House Staff; The President's Commission on the Health Needs of the Nation: Building America's Health* (GPO, 1951); Bernard J. Stern, *American Medical Practice* (New York: Commonwealth Fund, 1960); HEW, *Health Resources Statistics, 1965* (GPO, 1965), also volume for 1972–1973; American Medical Association, *Distribution of Physicians in the United States* (Chicago: AMA, 1965), 1; Walter Wiggins et al., "Medical Education in the United States," *Journal of the American Medical Association* 178 (November 11, 1961); American Medical Association, *Distribution of Physicians in the United States, 1970* (Chicago: AMA, 1971).

UNITED KINGDOM

House of Commons Papers, 1918, *Medical Education in England,* cmd. 9124, vol. 19; Robert Pinker, *English Hospital Statistics, 1861–1938* (London: Heinemann, 1966); Rosemary Stevens, *Medical Practice in Modern*

England: The Impact of Specialization and State Medicine (New Haven: Yale University Press, 1966); Arthur Newsholme, *International Studies on the Relation between the Private and Official Practice of Medicine* (London: Allen and Unwin, 1931), vol. 3; Political and Economic Planning, *Report on the British Health Services: A Survey of the Existing Health Services in Great Britain with Prospects for Future Development* (London: PEP, 1937); Brian Abel-Smith, *The Hospitals, 1800–1948* (London: Heinemann, 1964); Arthur Newsholme, *The Ministry of Health* (London: G. P. Putnam's Sons, 1925); annual reports of MOH, *Health and Personal Services Statistics; The Third Report on Metropolitan Hospitals* (HMSO, 1892); MOH, *Hospitals Survey* (HMSO, 1945).

FRANCE

Arthur Newsholme, *International Studies on the Relation between the Private and Office Practice of Medicine* (London: Allen and Unwin, 1935), vol. 2; American Medical Association, *The French Health Care System* (Chicago: AMA, 1976); Barbara Armstrong, *The Health Insurance Doctor: His Role in Great Britain, Denmark, and France* (Princeton: Princeton University Press, 1939); William Glaser, *Paying the Doctor: Systems of Remuneration and Their Effects* (Baltimore: Johns Hopkins University Press, 1970); James Hogarth, *The Payment of the General Practitioner: Some European Comparisons* (London: Pergamon Press, 1963); Alan Maynard, *Health Care in the European Community* (Pittsburgh: University of Pittsburgh Press, 1975); *ASF*; Ministère de la Santé Publique et de la Sécurité Sociale, *Bulletin de statistique*, no. 1 (January–February 1972); François Steudler, "Le systeme hospitalier: Evolution et transformation" (Ph.D diss., Centre d'Etude des Mouvements Sociaux, Paris, 1973); Henri Hatzfeld, Du pauperisme a la sécurité sociale: Essai sur les origines de la sécurité sociale en France, 1850–1940 (Paris: Armand Collin, 1971); Laurence C. Thorsen, "How Can the U.S. Government Control Physician's Fees under National Health Insurance? A Lesson from the French System", *International Journal of Health Services* 4 (May 1974), 49–57.

SWEDEN

SA; Ole Berg, "The Modernization of Medical Care in Sweden and Norway," in Arnold J. Heidenheimer and Nils Elvander, eds., *The Shaping of the Swedish Health System* (New York: St. Martin's Press, 1980); Hirobumi Ito, "Health Insurance and Medical Services in Sweden and Denmark, 1850–1950," ibid.

Sources for Table 2.3

UNITED STATES

For 1910–1920, extrapolation from *HSUS*; 1930–1970, *HSUS*.

Henry C. Burdett, *Burdett's Hospitals and Charities* (London: Scientific Press, 1914, 1921, 1930); *Forty-third Annual Report of the Local Government Board, 1913–1914,* Supplement containing Report of the Medical Officer, cmd. 7612 (HMSO, 1914); Arthur Newsholme, *International Studies on the Relation between the Private and Official Practice of Medicine* (London: Allen and Unwin, 1931); Robert Pinker, *English Hospital Statistics, 1861–1938* (London: Heinemann, 1966); *Report of the Local Government Board,* cmd. 6327 (HMSO, 1912); *Report of the Royal Commission on the Poor Laws and Relief of Distress,* vol. 25, Statistical Appendix, cmd. 4499 (HMSO, 1909); "Return as to the Administration of Sanatorium Benefits from January 12, 1914, to December 31, 1914," cmd. 8845 (HMSO, 1917); Royal Commission on the Poor Laws and Relief of Distress, *Report on Scotland,* cmd. 4922 (HMSO, 1909); Royal Commission on the Poor Laws and Relief of Distress, *Report on Scotland (Statistical and Other Documents Relating Specially to Scotland)* vol. 30, Appendix, cmd. 5440 (HMSO, 1911); *Seventeenth Annual Report of the Local Government Board for Scotland,* cmd. 6192 (HMSO, 1911); MOH, *Annual Reports, 1920–1921, 1921–1922, 1922–1923, 1931–1932; Third Annual Report of the Scottish Board of Health, 1921,* cmd. 1697 (HMSO, 1922); Government of Northern Ireland, *Report of the Ministry of Home Affairs on the Administration of Local Government Services for the Period from 1st December 1921 to 31st March 1923,* cmd. 30 (Belfast: HMSO, 1924); *The Hospitals Yearbook* (London: N.p., 1931, 1933, 1952, 1963, 1973); *The Annual Report of the Chief Medical Officer of the Ministry of Health, 1933, 1932; Annual Report of the Department of Health for Scotland,* cmd. 4080 (HMSO, 1932); Government of Northern Ireland, Ministry of Home Affairs, *The Administration of Local Government Services, 1935–1936,* cmd. 181 (HMSO, 1937); Great Britain, Department of Health and Social Security, *Health and Personal Social Services Statistics, 1972* (HMSO, 1973).

These sources were also used for Table 2.6. Data for the earlier years were more problematic, and it was necessary to augment the basic data found in Burdett. Estimates could be made on the basis of existing or partial data for 1891, 1921, 1938, 1961, and 1971. For 1901, 1931, and 1951 graphing and interpolation were used.

The same data sources are used for Tables 2.3 and 2.6: public hospital data from *ASF*; private hospital data, 1952–1971, from *ASF*; private hospital data, 1891–1951, estimated on the basis of change in public hospital sector. Retrospective data for the private sector was published in *ASF* in 1951, for a limited number of years. Using this and other sources indicating the age of institutional stock, the authors estimated the size of the private sector at different times.

SWEDEN

The same data sources were used for Tables 2.3 and 2.6: *SA*, 1932, 1945, 1953, 1962, 1972.

Sources for Table 2.4

Recent estimates of total medical system costs vary widely, and little systematic material has been available for the period before World War II. We have attempted to capture expenditure on all medical treatments. Where possible we have included expenditures for all drugs (not just those dispensed on prescription through pharmacists) and payments to all medical practitioners (including midwives, chiropractors, herbalists, healers, and the like).

UNITED STATES

The Statutes at Large of the United States of America from December 1889 to March 1891, vol. 26 (GPO, 1891); *Eleventh Decennial Census of the United States*, vol. 15: *Wealth, Debt and Taxation*, pt. 2; *Sixth Annual Report of the U.S. Commissioner of Labor for 1890; Seventh Annual Report of the U.S. Commissioner of Labor for 1891; HSUS; Eighteenth Annual Report of the U.S. Commissioner of Labor for 1903;* HEW, Social Security Administration, Office of Research and Statistics, by Barbara S. Cooper, Nancy L. Worthington, and Mary F. McGee, *Compendium of National Health Expenditures Data* (1976).

UNITED KINGDOM

Henry C. Burdett, *Burdett's Hospitals and Charities* (London: Scientific Press, 1914, 1921, 1933); Great Britain, Local Government Board, *Forty-third Annual Report of the Local Government Board, 1913–1914*, Supplement containing the report of the medical officer, cmd. 7612 (HMSO, 1914); Arthur Newsholme, *International Studies on the Relation between the Private and Official Practice of Medicine* (London: Allen and Unwin, 1931; Robert Pinker, *English Hospital Statistics, 1861–1938* (London: Heinemann, 1966); Great Britain, Local Government Board, *Report of the Local Government Board*, cmd. 6327 (HMSO, 1912); Great Britain, Royal Commission on the Poor Laws and Relief of Distress, *Report*, vol. 25: *Statistical Appendix*, cmd. 4499 (HMSO, 1909); Great Britain, "Return as to the Administration of Sanatorium Benefit from January 12, 1914, to December 31, 1914," cmd. 8834 (HMSO, 1917); Great

Britain, Royal Commission on the Poor Laws and Relief of Distress, *Report on Scotland*, cmd. 4922 (HMSO, 1909); Great Britain, Royal Commission on the Poor Laws and Relief of Distress, *Report on Scotland (Statistical and Other Documents Relating Specifically to Scotland)*, appendix, cmd. 5440 (HMSO, 1911); Great Britain, Local Government Board, *Seventeenth Annual Report of the Local Government Board for Scotland*, cmd. 6192 (HMSO, 1911); MOH, *Second Annual Report, 1920–1921*, cmd. 1146 (HMSO, 1921); MOH, *Third Annual Report, 1921–1922* (HMSO, 1922); MOH, *Annual Report, 1922–1923* (HMSO, 1923); *EHS*; Great Britain, Scottish Board of Health, *Third Annual Report of the Scottish Board of Health, 1921*, cmd. 1697 (HMSO, 1922); Government of Northern Ireland, *Report of the Ministry of Home Affairs on the Administration of Local Government Services for the Period from 1st December 1921 to 31st March 1923*, cmd. 30 (Belfast: HMSO, 1924); Central Bureau of Hospital Information, *The Hospitals Yearbook* (London: Central Bureau of Hospital Information, 1933); MOH, *The Annual Report of the Chief Medical Officer of the Ministry of Health for the Year 1933 on the State of Public Health*, (HMSO, 1934); MOH, *Chief Medical Officer's Report for 1932*, cmd. 4113 (HMSO, 1932); MOH, *Ministry of Health Report, 1931–1932* (HMSO); MOH, *Thirteenth Annual Report* (HMSO); Great Britain, *Annual Report of the Department of Health for Scotland*, cmd. 4080 (HMSO, 1932); Government of Northern Ireland, Ministry of Home Affairs, *The Administration of Local Government Services, 1935–1936*, cmd. 181 (Belfast: HMSO, 1937); Odin W. Anderson, *Health Care: Can There Be Equity?* (New York: John Wiley, 1972); Great Britain, Central Office of Information, *Health Services in Britain* (London: Central Office of Information, 1974); Great Britain, Central Statistical Office, *Annual Abstract of Statistics, 1973* (HMSO, 1973); Parliament of Northern Ireland, *Summary of Health Services Accounts, 1960–1961* (Belfast: HMSO, 1971); Great Britain, Department of Health and Social Security, *Health and Personal Social Services Statistics for England and Wales (with Summary Tables for Great Britain), 1972* (HMSO, 1973); A. R. Prest and A. A. Adams, eds., *Studies in the National Income and Expenditure of the United Kingdom*, vol. 3: *Consumer's Expenditure in the United Kingdom, 1900–1919* (Cambridge: Cambridge University Press, 1954); Richard Stone and D. A. Rowe, eds., *Studies in the National Income and Expenditure of the United Kingdom*, vol. 2: *The Measurement of Consumers' Expenditure and Behavior in the United Kingdom, 1920–1938* (Cambridge: Cambridge University Press, 1954); Bentley B. Gilbert, *The Evolution of National Insurance in Great Britain: The Origins of the Welfare State* (London: Joseph, 1966); R. W. Harris, *National Health Insurance in Great Britain, 1911–1946* (London: Allen and Unwin, 1946); United Kingdom, Central Statistical Office, *Statistical Abstract of the United Kingdom* (HMSO, various years); Charles Booth, *Life and Labor of the People in London* (New York: AMS Press, 1970).

FRANCE

Seventh Annual Report of the Commissioner of Labor, 1891: Cost of Production: Textiles and Glass, vol 2, pt. 3: *The Cost of Living* (GPO, 1892); J. Marczewski, "The Take-off Hypothesis and the French Experience," in W. W. Rostow, ed., *The Economics of Take-Off into Sustained Growth* (New York: St. Martin's Press, 1965); *ASF*; Pierre Theil, "Ce que la santé publique et le corps médical doivent a la sécurité sociale," *Les annales de médecine practicienne et sociale*, no. 147, 148, and 149 (March–May 1956). Figures for 1890–1930, checked against Henry Berenger, *Les prolétaires intellectuals en France* (Paris: Ancienne Revue des Revues, 1901); H. Cloyet, "Le budget ouvrière au temps présent," *Réforme Sociale* 87 (1927): 145–56; Maurice Halwachs, "Budgets de familles ouvrières et paysannes en France en 1907," *Bulletin Statistique Général de la France* 4:47–83; Jules Houdoy, *La filature de coton dans le nord de la France* (Paris: Librairie Nouvelle de Droit et de Jurisprudence, 1903); Louis Roussel, "Monographie d'une famille ouvrière de Lorraine," *Réforme Sociale* 88 (1928): 289–320; *Statistique Generale: Statistique d'institutions d'assistance* (IN, 1888, 1901, 1911, 1921, 1931); Ministère du Travail, *Rapport sur les orpérations des sociétés de secours mutuels pendant l'année 1910* (Paris: Ministère du Travail, 1913); François Perroux, "Prise de vues sur la croissance de l'économie française, 1780–1950," *Income and Wealth*, ser. 5; Maurice Rochaix, *Essai sur l'évolution des questions Hospitalières* (Paris: Fédération Hospitalière de France, 1959); Georges Rösch, *Economique médicale: Un système de services collectifs* (Paris: Flammarion Médecine-Sciences, 1973); Georges Rösch, "L'économie des services de soins médicaux en France," *Consommation* 15.2 (Paris: Centre de Recherches et de Documentation sur la Consommation, April–June 1969); Albert Palmberg, *L'hygiene publique en France* (Paris: Ministère de Santé, 1930); Pierre Laroque, ed., *Social Welfare in France* (Paris: Documentation Française, 1966).

SWEDEN

Medicinalstyrelsen, *Allman halso-och sjukvard, 1920*, also 1930, 1940, 1944, 1950, 1960, 1965, and 1970; Socialstyrelsen, *Sociala meddelanden*, ser. F, vol. 29 (Stockholm: Norstedt, 1926); Statistiska Centralbyran, *Folkrakningen den 31 december 1920*, also 1930, 1945, and 1970 (Stockholm: Norstedt); Statistiska Centralbyran, *Kommunernas finanser*, 1925, 1942, and 1972; *SA* 1933, 1945; Odin Anderson, *Health Care: Can There Be Equity?* (New York: John Wiley, 1972); Stephen Hammerqvist, "Economy and Health Personnel—Determining Issues in the Swedish

Health Delivery System" (Unpublished paper presented to the International Conference on Changing National-Subnational Relations in Health, May 24–26, 1976); Riksforsakringsverket, *Allman forsakring ar 1970* (Stockholm: Allman Forlaget, 1972); Socialstyrelsen, *RUPRO, 1971* (Stockholm: Socialstyrelsen, 1971); Erik Lindahl, Einar Dahlgren, and Karin Kock, *National Income of Sweden, 1861–1930* (Stockholm: Institute for Social Sciences, 1937). Data for earlier time points were extrapolated.

Sources for Table 2.5

UNITES STATES

Data on physicians from *HSUS*, 1890–1970; also United States Decennial Census, 1890, *Compendium*; United States Decennial Census, 1900, *Special Report on Occupations;* United States Decennial Census, 1930, *Population;* United States Decennial Census, 1950, *Population;* HEW, *The Supply of Health Manpower, 1962;* HEW, *Health Resources Statistics, 1971, 1974. HSUS* was used to estimate, for the early years, the number of trained, as opposed to self-declared, doctors. For 1980, Organization for Economic Cooperation and Development, *Measuring Health Care, 1960–1983: Expenditure, Costs, and Performance* (Paris: OECD Social Policy Studies, no. 2, 1985), 90, 154, was used for all four countries. For specialists, we used the above data in conjunction with Rosemary Stevens, *American Medicine and the Public Interest* (New Haven: Yale University Press, 1971), to interpret both physician and specialist data, correcting data for desired years.

UNITED KINGDOM

Data on physicians from *Census of England and Wales,* for 1891, 1901, 1911, 1921; *Tenth Decennial Census of Scotland, 1891; Eleventh Decennial Census of Scotland, 1901; Twelfth Decennial Census of Scotland, 1911; Report of the Thirteenth Decennial Census of Scotland; Census of England and Wales, 1931: Occupation Tables; Report on the Fourteenth Decennial Census of Scotland,* vol. 3: *Occupations and Industries; Census, 1951: England and Wales County Reports; Census of Scotland, 1951,* vol. 4: *Occupations and Industries.* We interpolated for England and Wales for 1941. Years 1951–1971 were estimated with reliance on *Census of Population of Northern Ireland General Report* (1955); *Census of Population, 1961, General Report* (for Northern Ireland, 1965); *Census of Population, 1971, General Report* (for Northern Ireland, 1975); *Health and Personal Social Services Statistics for England and Wales, 1972; Health Services in Scotland: Reports for 1971; Annual Abstracts of Statistics, 1973.* Estimates of specialists were based on *Health and Personal Social Services Statistics for England*

and Wales, 1972, adjusted with reference to Rosemary Stevens, *Medical Practice in Modern England: The Impact of Specialization and State Medicine* (New Haven: Yale University Press, 1966); and Odin Anderson, *Health Care: Can There Be Equity?* (New York: John Wiley, 1972). Data for 1891–1921 were based on above data sources and extrapolations.

FRANCE

Data on physicians, *ASF*, 1913, 1932, 1951, 1952, 1962, 1973; *Recueil de la Statistique,* vols. 39–42 (1943); Statistique Générale, *Statistiques du personnel médicale pour 1911* (1913); Statistique Générale, *Recensement de la population, 1891, 1896, 1901, 1911, 1921, 1931*; Ministère de l'Éducation, *Recueil de la statistique, 1949 à 1951* (1952). Estimates of specialists for 1911, 1921, 1931, and 1939 were derived from the percentage of Paris physicians advertising a recognized specialty in 1948. The figures, from the *Guide Rosenwald,* were adjusted for the whole of France. For 1951–1971, we used the data on physicians. See also Jean Bui-Ha-Doan and Daniele R. Levy, "Le rythme des qualifications de spécialistes et compétents jusqu'en 1966," *Cahiers de Sociologie et de Demographie Médicales* 7 (1967): 15–19. Data for 1891, 1901, 1941 were estimated by graphing, extrapolation, and interpolation.

SWEDEN

For physicians, Statistisk Centralbyran, *Folkrakningen den 31 december 1910* (also parallel census materials for 1920 and 1930); *SA* 1945, 1951, 1962, 1972. On specialists, data for 1900, 1920, 1940, from Swedish Institute, *Public Health and Medicine in Sweden* (Stockholm: Forum); for 1960, from Socialstyrelsen, *Allman halso-och sjukvard ar 1960* (Stockholm, 1962); for 1970, from Socialstyrelsen, *Allman halso-och sjukvard ar 1970* (Stockholm, 1972); for 1890, 1910, 1930, 1950, from interpolations and extrapolations from sources for other decades.

Sources for Table 2.6

UNITED STATES

American Medical Association, "Hospital Service in the United States," *Journal of the American Medical Association* (April 16, 1921, March 23, 1931, May 12, 1951), and data interpolated for 1910; American Hospital Association, "Hospital Statistics," *Journal of the American Hospital Association (June 15, 1951, August 1, 1961, August 1, 1971).*

UNITED KINGDOM, FRANCE, AND SWEDEN

Sources same as for Table 2.3.

Sources for Table 2.7

In order to control for inflation/deflation in gross national product, deflators were applied to the series from each country. The deflators were drawn from *EHS* and from Henry Phelps Brown and Margaret H. Browne, *A Century of Pay* (New York: St. Martin's, 1968). GNPs were further standardized by conversion into 1938 United States dollars, using currency relationships found in *Whitaker's Almanac, 1938* (London: Whitaker and Sons, 1937).

UNITED STATES

HSUS, 1900–1970 (data on communications for 1890 extrapolated); *Statistical Abstract of the United States*, 1960–1970; *Compendium of the U.S. Census, 1890*, vol. 3; *Census of the United States*, 1900 (*Population*, pt. 2), 1910 (*Population*, pt. 1), 1920 (vol. 2), 1930 (*Population*, vol. 2), 1940, 1950, 1960 (state vols.), 1970 (state population characteristics vols.).

UNITED KINGDOM

EHS (data on communication for 1900, 1910 estimated from partial *EHS* data); Central Statistical Office, *Annual Abstract of Statistics, 1971* (HMSO, 1971); Great Britain *Decennial Census*, 1891–1971; Great Britain *Registrar General Reports*, 1891–1971; *Parliamentary Papers*, 1893 ("The Brice Commission Report"), 1892 (28:ix, xxxiii), 1901 (vol. 19), 1912–1913 (vol. 64), 1938–1939 (vol. 10), 1951–1952 (vol. 10); *Board of Education Report, 1923*, cmd. 1896; *Census of England and Wales, 1921: Private Schools and Other Schools Not in Receipt of Grants from Public Funds* ("Chuter Ede Report") (HMSO, 1932); Grace G. Leybourne and Kenneth White, *Education and the Birth Rate: A Social Dilemma* (London: Jonathan Cape, 1940); *Parliamentary Report*, 1931–1932 (vol. 9); Department of Education and Science, *Statistics of Education, 1972*, vol. 1; J. A. C. Griffiths, *General Departments and Local Authorities* (Toronto: University of Toronto Press, 1966). Data on the number of local education authorities are taken from annual reports of the Ministry of Education and the Department of Education and Science. The precise number of wholly independent schools before 1951 is not known.

FRANCE

EHS (data for communications in 1890 extrapolated); *ASF* (data on the elderly for 1951 interpolated from *ASF*, 1936 and 1954); *Recensement générale de la population*, 1921, vol. 2; *ASF: Résumé retrospectif*, 1951, 1966; Maurice Lévy-Leboyer, "Le croissance l'économique en France au XIXe siècle: Résultats préliminaires," *Annales Economies-Sociétés-Civilisations* 23. 4 (1968); *Statistiques des écoles primaires* (IN: Ministère de l'Éducation, 1891, 1901, 1906, 1911); *Statistiques de l'enseignement secondaire en 1887* (IN); *Journal officiel: documents parlementaires, Chambre des Députés*, 7e législature, session de 1899, #866 (Paris: Imprimière de la Chambre des Députés), vol. 3, also 1909, #2757 (IN); *Recueil des statistiques* (Paris: Ministère de l'Éducation, 1936, 1941–43, 1949–51); *Information statistiques* (Paris: Ministère de l'Éducation, various years after 1957).

SWEDEN

EHS (data for communications in 1890 extrapolated); *SA; Sveriges officiella statistik sammandrag*, 1890–1910; *Folkrakningen*, 1920, 1930, 1940, 1950, 1960, 1970; *Befolkningsforandringar*, 1970. Because of the many types of schools and the lack of specific information as to the ages of students in Sweden, it was necessary to work extensively with the data collected. Our major sources were *Folkskolorna ar 1911; SA; Folkskolorna och hogre folkskolorna redovisningsaret, 1919–1920; Lararutbildningen lasaret, 1910–1921; Yrkesundervisningen aren, 1919–1921; De kommunala mellanskolorna lasaret, 1919–1920;* and Statens allmanmna laroverk ar 1921.

Sources for Table 4.1

UNITED STATES

United States Bureau of the Census, HEW, *Vital Statistics of the United States*, annual reports; United States Bureau of the Census, *Report on Vital and Social Statistics in the United States at the Eleventh Census*, pt. 1 (1896); United States Bureau of the Census, *Census Reports*, 1900, vol. 3.

UNITED KINGDOM

Great Britain, Office of Population Census and Surveys, *Decennial Census*, 1891–1971 (HMSO); Great Britain, *Registrar General Reports*, 1891–1971, 1978 (HMSO).

FRANCE

Statistique Général, *Statistique général de la France, 1890* (IN); Statistique Général, *Résultes statistiques du dénombrement de 1891* (IN, 1894); Statistique Général, *Mouvement de la population, 1899–1900, 1907–1913, 1914–1925, 1931, 1938* (adjusted to estimate 1940); *1951–1952, 1960–1962, 1965–1966* (IN); Statistique Général, *Résultes statistiques du recensement général de la population* (IN, 1901, 1911, 1921, 1931); Statistique Général, *Résultes statistique de la population, 1936* (adjusted to estimate 1940); Statistique Général, *Recensement général de la population, 1946;*

Statistique Général, *Recensement de la Population, 1954* (data for 1951 estimated from both these sources), *1954, 1962, 1968.*

SWEDEN

Sveriges officiella statistik i sammandrag (1896, 1906); *Sveriges officiella statistiska: Folksmangden och dess forandringar, folkrakningen den 31 december 1910,* vol. 2; *Folksrakningen den 31 december 1920,* vol. 3; *Folkrakningen den 31 december 1930,* vol. 2; *Folkrakningen den 31 december 1940,* vol. 2; *Folkrakningen den 31 december 1950,* vol. 5; *Folkrakningen den 1 november 1960,* vol. 3; *Befolkningsforandringar 1970,* vol. 3.

Appendix 2

INDEX CONSTRUCTION

In chapters 3–6 several multiple-variable indexes are used to represent the complex concepts of social development, state revenue control, and state price and personnel control. The construction of these indexes from the raw data was a somewhat complicated process.

The Social Development Index

The social development index is composed of four indicators, reflecting three different dimensions of modernization and development. The level of educational attainment of the population and levels of communication form one dimension, the age structure of the population the second, and the level of real material production per capita the third. The three dimensions were given equal weight in composing the summed index of social development.

Educational development and communication were taken as two indicators of societal modernization. Educational development was measured as the percentage of age-eligible population enrolled in secondary schools twenty years prior to each time point (that is, the index values for 1930 reflect enrollment rates in 1910). The level of communication was measured by the number of telephone conversations per capita for the year in question. To give each of these components equal weight, they were normalized by subtracting their means (calculated across all nations and time points) and dividing by their standard deviations. This procedure results in scores with means of zero and standard deviations of one. Each of these components was then given a weight of .5 in the final social development index. That is, since there were two indicators of the modernization dimension and only one indicator each for age structure and material production, education and communication were each given half the weight of these indicators.

The age structure of the population was measured as the ratio of the number of persons sixty-five or more years of age to the total population at each year in question. These scores were also normalized by subtracting the mean and dividing by the standard deviation of their distribution over the countries and time. The resulting normalized variable received a weight of one in the final social development index.

Finally, the level of material wealth was measured as the real (deflated) gross national product per capita, converted to 1938 U.S. dollars at average market exchange rates between the relevant currencies in each year. The year 1938 was chosen as a baseline for convenience, as it falls near the middle of the time period we are examining. The values of this variable were also normalized by subtracting the mean and dividing by the standard deviation pooled across nations and time. The resulting normalized variable received a weight of one in the final social development index.

The final social development index was constructed by adding together the weighted and normalized scores of the four indicators (education, communication, age structure, and real GNP). The purpose of the weighting and normalization is to provide each of the three dimensions (modernization, age structure, and material production) equal weight. The final values of the social development index have been linearly rescaled for presentational ease. The values reported range between zero, representing the lowest observed score, and one, representing the highest observed score.

Index of State Control over Revenues

Centralization under the auspices of the state, by means of control over system revenue, is measured using data on the sources of funding for medical treatment. For each observation (that is, nation-year), data were collected on the proportions of system revenues contributed by central government and social insurance authorities, local and regional government authorities, and private-sector actors. These proportions were weighted five, three, and one, respectively, and then summed.

The particular weights chosen are somewhat arbitrary, for the relative numbers of authorities within the central governments, local governments, and private sectors vary considerably across both nations and time. Nonetheless, the resulting index appropriately gives considerably greater weight to the capacities of governmental actors, and particularly to central authorities. Several alternative weights were explored but resulted in little substantive change in statistical results.

The values resulting from this procedure could vary, logically, between five, indicating that all revenues were controlled by central authorities to one, indicating that all revenues were controlled in the private sector. For ease of presentation, however, these values were linearly rescaled by subtracting one (to set the minimum value of the index to zero) and dividing by four (to set the maximum value to one).

Index of State Control over Prices and Personnel

Centralization under the auspices of the state by means of control over the appointment of personnel and the setting of prices is measured using data on the employment of physicians and expenditures in the medical care system.

The personnel centralization index is constructed from data on the proportion of physicians employed by central government and social insurance authorities, local government authorities, and private authorities (including self-employment) for each nation and year. These proportions, like the index of revenue control, are given weights of five, three, and one (for central government, local government, and private sectors) and then summed. This component of the index was then linearly rescaled to range between zero (all physicians employed in the private sector) and one (all physicians employed by central government authorities).

The index of price control was constructed in a similar fashion, using data on the proportions of all expenditures in the medical care system that occurred at prices regulated by central authorities, local authorities, and mechanisms of the private sector. These proportions were again weighted and linearly rescaled, as described previously, to vary between zero, indicating completely private control, to one, indicating total central governmental control.

In the data analyses reported in Chapters 3–6, the price and personnel indexes are combined into a single score. Since the two series have somewhat unequal variances (calculated across the pool of both nations and time), they have been normalized prior to being summed to create a single "price-personnel" index. This procedure has the effect of giv-

ing each of the component parts equal weight. The final values of the
price and personnel control index have been linearly rescaled for presentational ease. The values reported range between zero, representing
the lowest observed score, and one, representing the highest observed
score.

Appendix 3

REGRESSION ANALYSIS

In several chapters we report the results of fitting simultaneous equation models to the data for the four nations. These models are presented in the form of hierarchical (recursive) structural equations, and "path analysis" has been used to analyze and present the results. This approach to modeling the effects of social development, delivery system structure, and state intervention on the several outcomes is widely used in the social sciences. Readers unfamiliar with the techniques can find good introductions in Pedhazur, 1982; Kenny, 1979; Duncan, 1975, and other texts on multivariate analysis.

As we have said, the performance of medical care delivery systems must be understood as the outcome of multiple causes operating simultaneously. Consequently, it is appropriate to use statistical control to hold constant or adjust for the effects of all the other independent variables to assess the magnitude of the effect of each independent variable on performance. In taking the further step of specifying the model as a hierarchical (recursive) system of simultaneous equations, we are also seeking insight into the indirect mechanisms by which changes in social development and delivery system structure operate to change performance. Imposing hierarchical order among the independent variables in the structural equations enables us to interpret the joint effects of independent variables that speak directly to our theories of the causal mechanisms connecting changes in social development,

delivery system structure, and state intervention on system performance.

Hierarchical structural equation models are used to interpret the
multivariate associations among variables precisely because they allow
examination of the direct and indirect effects of independent variables
in light of theories about causal processes. For such interpretations to
be valid, however, a number of conditions must be satisfied. First, all
the routine statistical assumptions underlying the use of linear regression analysis (most notably the linearity of relationships and the nor-
mality of distributions) must be met. Second, care must be taken that
the hierarchical ordering of the variables is justified. Third, special
problems arise in the proper estimation of effects when the data used
are drawn from a pooled cross-sectional and time-series design, as is
the case in the current analysis.

The first two conditions have been relatively easy to satisfy. Graphic
examination of the bivariate and multivariate relationships, as well as
diagnosis of the residuals from regressions, suggests that the data are
well conditioned in these regards. In some cases, logarithmic transformations have been used both to linearize relationships and to homoge-
nize variances. The questions of the proper specification of causal order and difficulties arising from using pooled cross sections and time
series, however, require somewhat lengthier discussion.

Specification of Causal Order

Imposing causal ordering on the independent variables by use of a hierarchical model is extremely desirable because it allows us to speak to
the issue of how changes in some independent variables operate indirectly through mediating variables to change system performance. For
such interpretations to be valid, however, there must be strong theoretical justification for the causal ordering of the variables. If, for example, our model specifies that variable A causes variable B, when, in
fact, variable B causes variable A (or A and B cause one another), we
are led into interpretational errors about the meaning of the joint associations between A and B and outcome variables.

The ordering of the variables in our models implies a series of theoretical assumptions. We assume that social development affects delivery
system structure, state intervention, and outcomes but is not affected
by them; that delivery system structure affects state intervention and
outcomes but is not affected by them; that state intervention in revenue
affects state intervention in price and personnel control as well as outcomes but is not affected by them; and that state intervention in price
and personnel matters affects outcomes but not vice versa.

A moment's reflection suggests that none of these assumptions is wholly warranted. The level of medical expenditure, state intervention, and system size and specialization do help to shape population age structures and even gross national product. State intervention has been used to modify physician supply and specialization on some occasions in some nations. Most obviously, levels of system performance are often part of the stimulus for change in physician supply, specialization, and state intervention. That is, in real systems (as opposed to our statistical model), causal arrows often run in both directions.

The estimation of fully simultaneous systems of equations with all possible feedbacks cannot be done with the current data (and is extremely difficult under any circumstances). Consequently, there is some danger that bias has resulted from our inability to take these feedback processes into account. The biases that result from failing to model these processes directly are false attribution to a given variable of effects that are, in fact, the result of complex feedbacks involving two or more variables. Such interpretational biases are proportional to the relative magnitudes of the true feedforward and feedback relationships. If omitted feedback effects are large and positive, the parameter estimates from our models will overstate the importance of an independent variable; if the omitted feedback effects are large and negative, our models will understate the true importance of an independent variable.

The causal ordering of variables specified in the model, then, can be quite important. We are convinced that our models approximate the more complex reality of the causes connecting societal conditions, delivery system structure, state intervention, and outcomes. Because our case for the models is strong, we are similarly convinced that the parameters of our statistical models are reasonably good approximations of the "true" magnitudes of the effects.

The largest part of our case for the proper specification of the statistical models lies in the theory and logic of the causal mechanisms involved. The large-scale societal changes measured by the social development index most certainly constrain the development of delivery system structure, state intervention, and medical outcomes. While these latter variables are consequential for gross national product, modernization, and age structures, the magnitudes of these feedback effects are relatively small (as shown, for example, by the limited effects of delivery system and state intervention variables on mortality rates, relative to the effects of social development). The feedback effects, to the limited extent that they operate, also operate much more slowly than the feedforward effects. Consequently, any upward bias in the effects of social development on the other variables shown in our models is likely to be very small. The relationships between delivery system structure, and outcomes are somewhat more problematic in terms of proper specification of causal order. We maintain, on the basis of our historical understanding of the development of these systems, that state intervention has a very strong tendency to be consequent to and shaped by delivery system structure, rather than the reverse. Similarly, our reading of the history of these systems compels the conclusion that state intervention has its own logic: significant interventions in financing of medical care precede intervention in direct regulation and management. Again, whereas feedback processes do exist, the predominant causal direction of the connections among the independent variables is clearly in the direction specified by our models.

The most important evidence about the proper causal ordering of variables must come from the plausibility of our theories about the magnitudes, directions, and speeds of causal mechanisms. Nevertheless, some statistical results speak to (but cannot resolve) the issue. In the relationship between delivery system structure and state intervention, on one hand, and outcome variables, on the other, it is notable that controls for delivery system structure variables do not markedly modify the effects of state intervention on outcomes. Controls for state intervention variables, however, do substantially reduce the unique or direct effects of delivery system variables on outcomes. This pattern is consistent with (but does not prove) the hypothesis that state intervention mediates the effects of delivery system variables on outcomes, rather than the opposite.

In sum, the causal ordering of variables in hierarchical structural equation models is quite important. Misspecification of ordering and excluding feedback relations can be important for the proper interpretation of parameter estimates. The logic of the theory, historical evidence, and statistical patterns all suggest that such specification problems are not likely to be a major threat to our conclusions about the relative magnitudes of direct and indirect effects of social development, delivery system structure, and state intervention on medical system performance.

Estimation Problems

The standard method of estimating the parameters of structural equation models (ordinary least squares, or OLS) which assumes that the observations are a random sample of some larger universe of observations, is suitable if one is seeking to explain the growth of wheat plants using levels of rainfall, fertilizer, and the like as independent variables. In such a case each stalk selected at random for measurement is in no way connected with the other stalks that could have been chosen. The data used for our analysis, however, do not satisfy the sampling assumption of independent observations. As a result, there is some reason for concern about the parameters estimated from the data by means of OLS.

There are two sources of nonindependence in the pooled time-series and cross-sectional data used to estimate the parameters of our models. First and most obvious, are the four groups of observations in the data set, one for each country. We might reasonably expect two observations from the same country to be more similar than two observations drawn at random. It is reasonable to expect that other factors aside from those explicitly included also affect the dependent variables in our models, and these omitted variables may differ from one nation to the next because of different history, culture, etc. Second, our observations form nine groups according to decade points, and factors other than the variables included in the model are causing trends within each nation. Again, there is reason to expect that the observations at any one time may resemble those from an adjacent time more than two observations drawn at random. Statistically, this situation results in "correlated errors," and such correlations may bias the magnitudes of the parameters. To assess the true causal influence of independent variables on dependent variables, these error components of the total variance due to pooling cross sections and time series should be removed from the calculations.

Preliminary analysis of our data for each nation by OLS identified a number of equations with significant Durbin-Watson tests for serially correlated error. In some cases, the estimated autoregressive parameters (rho) were larger than .50. The presence of error correlations of this magnitude suggested that OLS estimates of the standard errors of coefficients could be substantially distorted, and that with relatively few observations the magnitudes of some coefficients could be overstated. Consequently, we have adopted an alternative Generalized Least Squares (GLS) method for the calculation of parameters that allows for the presence of certain kinds of correlated errors.

Unfortunately, there is no single, generally accepted method for dealing with the problems of the error structures of pooled cross sections and time series. Substantial research has been devoted to the question over the years (Kuh, 1959; Balestra and Nerlove, 1966; Wallace and Hussain, 1969; Maddala, 1971; Nerlove, 1971; Kmenta, 1986). More recently, useful computer programs allow one to calculate the parameters of such models under alternative sets of assumptions about the structures of the error components (Drummond and Gallant, 1979).

The most appropriate error components model for the data used in Chapters 2, 3, 4, and 6 is one proposed by Parks (cited in Drummond and Gallant, 1979). Drummond and Gallant state, "The Parks method assumes a first-order autoregressive error structure with contemporaneous correlation between cross-sections." That is, the model allows for the possibility that errors are serially correlated within each nation, and that there may be systematic components of the errors in all nations for particular years. Thus, the regression coefficients reported in the various figures and tables in these chapters are those calculated by the Parks GLS method. Because this method is not appropriate to analyze the data in Chapter 5, we used the OLS method in that chapter.

Virtually all statistical models in the social sciences need to be appreciated with proper caution for specification, sampling design, and measurement concerns. The results reported herein are no exception to this rule. We believe, however, that our results are quite robust against the most common difficulties that arise in problems of the type considered here. Thus, although they should hardly be taken as the final word on the questions of this research, they do constitute substantial evidence in favor of the conclusions we have reached. Moreover, we have gone to great lengths to employ qualitative methods and data to complement the quantitative analysis. We believe that both quantitative and qualitative methods strongly buttress the arguments developed in this book.

BIBLIOGRAPHY

Aaron, Henry J., and William B. Schwartz. 1984. *The Painful Prescription: Rationing Hospital Care* (Washington, D.C.: Brookings Institution).

Abel-Smith, Brian. 1963. "Paying for Health Services," *Public Health Papers* 17 (Geneva: World Health Organization).

Abel-Smith, Brian. 1964. *The Hospitals, 1800–1948* (London: Heinemann).

Abel-Smith, Brian. 1965. "The Major Pattern of Financing and the Organization of Medical Services That Have Emerged in Other Countries," *Medical Care* 3 (January–March): 33–40.

Abel-Smith, Brian. 1967. "An International Study of Health Expenditure," *Public Health Papers* 32 (Geneva: World Health Organization).

Abel-Smith, Brian. 1969. "Etude internationale des dépenses de santé: Leur incidence sur la planification des services médico-sanitaires," *Cahiers de Santé Publique* 32.

Abel-Smith, Brian. 1976. *Value for Money in Health Services* (London: Heinemann).

Abel-Smith, Brian, and Richard Titmuss. 1956. *The Cost of the National Health Service in England and Wales* (Cambridge: Cambridge University Press).

Abt Associates. 1975. *Incentives and Decisions underlying Hospitals' Adoption and Utilization of Major Capital Equipment* (Boston: N.p.).

Ackerknecht, Erwin H. 1945. *Malaria in the Upper Mississippi Valley, 1760–1900* (Baltimore: Johns Hopkins University Press).

Ackerknecht, Erwin H. 1957. "Medical Education in 19th Century France," *Journal of Medical Education* 32 (February): 148–53.

Ackerknecht, Erwin H. 1967. *Medicine at the Paris Hospitals, 1798–1848* (Baltimore: Johns Hopkins University Press).

Aday, LuAnn, Ronald Andersen, and Gretchen V. Fleming. 1980. *Health Care in the U.S.: Equitable for Whom?* (Beverly Hills, Calif.: Sage).

Aiken, Michael, and Robert Alford. 1970. "Community Structure and Innovation: The Case of Public Housing," *American Political Science Review* 64 (September): 843–65.

Aiken, Michael, and Jerald Hage. 1966. "Organizational Alienation: A Comparative Analysis," *American Sociological Review* 31 (August): 497–507.

Aiken, Michael, and Jerald Hage. 1968. "Organizational Interdependence and Intraorganizational Structure," *American Sociological Review* 33: 912–30.

Aiken, Michael, and Jerald Hage. 1971. "The Organic Organization and Innovation," *Sociology* 5: 63–82.

Aldrich, Howard E. 1979. *Organizations and Environments* (Englewood Cliffs, N.J.: Prentice-Hall).

Alford, Robert R. 1975. *Health Care Politics: Ideological and Interest Group Barriers to Reform* (Chicago: University of Chicago Press).

Alford, Robert R., and Roger Friedland. 1985. *Powers of Theory: Capitalism, the State, and Democracy* (Cambridge: Cambridge University Press).

Almond, Gabriel A., and G. Bingham Powell, Jr. 1966. *Comparative Politics: A Developmental Approach* (Boston: Little, Brown).

American Medical Association. 1976. *The French Health Care System* (Chicago: American Medical Association).

Andersen, Ronald, Bjorn Smedby, and Odin W. Anderson. 1970. *Medical Care Use in Sweden and the United States—A Comparative Analysis of Systems and Behavior*, R.S. no. 27 (Chicago: Center for Health Administration Studies).

Andersen, Ronald, et al. 1976. *Two Decades of Health Services: Social Survey Trends in Use and Expenditure* (Cambridge, Mass.: Ballinger).

Anderson, Odin W. 1968. *The Uneasy Equilibrium: Private and Public Financing of Health Services in the United States, 1875–1965* (New Haven, Conn.: College and University Press).

Anderson, Odin W. 1972. *Health Care: Can There Be Equity? The United States, Sweden, and England* (New York: John Wiley).

Anderson, Odin W., and James Warner Bjorkman. 1980. "Equity and Health Care: Sweden, Britain, and the United States," in Arnold Heidenheimer and Nils Elvander, eds., *The Shaping of the Swedish Health System* (New York: St. Martin's Press), 223–37.

Anton, Thomas J. 1969. "Policy Making and Political Culture in Sweden," *Scandinavian Political Studies* 4: 88–102.

Aoki, Masahiko. 1988. *Information, Incentives, and Bargaining in the Japanese Economy* (Cambridge: Cambridge University Press).

Apple, Rima. 1987. *Mothers and Medicine: A Social History of Infant Feeding, 1890–1950* (Madison: University of Wisconsin Press).

Appleby, A. B. 1975. "Nutrition and Disease: The Case of London, 1550–1750," *Journal of Interdisciplinary History* 6: 1–22.

Archer, Margaret. 1982. *The Sociology of Educational Expansion: Take-off, Growth, and Inflation in Educational Systems* (Beverly Hills: Sage).

Auster, Richard, Irving Leveson, and Deborah Sarachek. 1969. "The Production of Health: An Exploratory Study," *Journal of Human Resources* 4 (Fall): 411–36.

Ayers, Gwendolyn. 1971. *England's First State Hospitals and the Metropolitan Asylums Board, 1867–1930* (London: Wellcome Institute of the History of Medicine).

Azumi, Koya, and Jerald Hage, eds. 1972. *Organizational Systems* (Lexington, Mass.: D. C. Heath).

Baker, Josephine S. 1913. "The Reduction of Infant Mortality in New York City," *American Journal of Diseases of Children* 5: 151–61.

Balestra, Pietro, and Marc Nerlove. 1966. "Pooling Cross-Section and Time-Series Data in the Estimation of a Dynamic Model: The Demand for Natural Gas," *Econometrica* 34: 585–612.

Banta, H. David. 1980. "The Diffusion of the Computer Tomography (CT) Scanner in the United States," *International Journal of Health Services* 10: 251–69.

Barnard, Chester. 1946. "Functions and Pathology of Status Systems in Formal Organizations," in William F. Whyte, ed., *Industry and Society* (New York: McGraw-Hill).

Barnett, Homer G. 1953. *Innovation* (New York: McGraw-Hill).

Beaver, M. W. 1973. "Population, Infant Mortality, and Milk," *Population Studies* 27 (July): 243–54.

Beck, R. G. 1974. "The Effects of Copayment on the Poor," *Journal of Human Resources* 9 (Winter): 129–42.

Becker, Gary. 1964. *Human Capital* (New York: National Bureau of Economic Research).

Becker, M. 1970. "Sociometric Location and Innovativeness: Reformulation and an Extension of the Diffusion Model," *American Sociological Review* 35 (April): 267–82.

Bell, Daniel. 1973. *The Coming of Post-industrial Society: A Venture in Social Forecasting* (New York: Basic Books).

Ben-David, Joseph. 1971. *The Scientist's Role in Society: A Comparative Study* (Englewood Cliffs, N.J.: Prentice-Hall).

Bendick, Marc, Jr. 1975. "Education as a Three-Sector Industry" (Ph.D. diss., University of Wisconsin, Madison).

Bendick, Marc, Jr. 1985. "Privatizing the Delivery of Social Welfare Services," *Working Paper No. 6: Privatization* (Washington, D.C.: National Conference on Social Welfare).

Berg, Ivar. 1970. *Education and Jobs: The Great Training Robbery* (New York: Praeger).

Berg, Ole. 1980. "The Modernization of Medical Care in Sweden and Norway," in Arnold J. Heidenheimer and Nils Elvander, ed., *The Shaping of the Swedish Health System* (New York: St. Martin's Press), 17–43.

Blackstone, Erwin A. 1977. "The Condition of Surgery: An Analysis of the American College of Surgeons and the American Surgical Association's Report on the Status of Surgery," *Milbank Memorial Fund Quarterly* 55 (Fall): 429–54.

Blake, Donald J. 1960. "Swedish Trade Unions and the Social Democratic Party: The Formative Years," *Scandinavian Economic History Review* 8: 19–44.

Blake, John B. 1948. "The Origins of Public Health in the United States," *American Journal of Public Health* 38 (November): 1539–50.

Blake, Nelson M. 1956. *Water for the Cities: A History of the Urban Water Supply Problem in the United States* (Syracuse, N.Y.: Syracuse University Press).

Blau, Peter M. 1970. "Decentralization in Bureaucracies," in Mayer N. Zald, ed., *Power in Organizations* (Nashville: Vanderbilt University Press).

Blau, Peter M. 1972. "Interdependence and Hierarchy in Organizations," *Social Science Research* 1 (April): 2– 24.

Blau, Peter M. 1973. *The Organization of Academic Work* (New York: John Wiley).

Blau, Peter M., and Richard Schoenherr. 1971. *The Structure of Organizations* (New York: Basic Books).

Boudon, Raymond. 1974. *Education, Opportunity, and Social Inequality* (New York: John Wiley).

Bowles, Samuel, and Herbert Gintis. 1976. *Schooling in Capitalist America* (New York: Basic Books).

Brand, Jeanne L. 1961. "The Parish Doctor: England's Poor Law Medical Officers and Medical Reform, 1870–1900," *Bulletin of the History of Medicine* 35: 97–122.

Brand, Jeanne L. 1965. *Doctors and the State: The British Medical Profession and Government Action in Public Health, 1870–1912* (Baltimore: Johns Hopkins University Press).

Braverman, Harry. 1974. *Labor and Monopoly Capital* (New York: Monthly Review Press).

Brems, Hans. 1970. "Sweden: From Great Power to Welfare State," *Journal of Economic Issues* 4.2–3: 1–17.

Brenner, M. Harvey. 1987. "Relations of Economic Change to Swedish Health and Social Well-Being, 1950–1980," *Social Science and Medicine* 25: 183–95.

Bridgman, R. F. 1971. "Medical Care under Social Security in France," *International Journal of Health Services* 1 (November): 331–41.

Brittan, Samuel. 1985. "The Politics and Economics of Privatization," *Political Quarterly* 55 (June): 109–28.

Broun, Georges. 1969. "Le financement des coûts de la maladie: Essai d'analyse économique," *Revue Française des Affaires Sociales* (January–March): 1–18.

Brown, Lawrence. 1978. "The Scope and Limits of Equality as a Normative Guide to Federal Health Care Policy," *Public Policy* 26 (Fall): 481–532.

Bugbee, George. 1958. "Comments on Government Medicine in England and France," *Journal of the American Medical Association* 166 (March 22): 1474–78.

Bui-Dang-Ha-Doan, J. 1970. "Evolutions récentes du corps médical français," *Cahiers de Sociologie et Démographie Médicale* (April–June): 83–93.

Bui-Dang-Ha-Doan, J., and Laurent Gwenaelle. 1970. "Structures actuelles de la profession médicale," *Cahiers de Sociologie et Démographie Médicale* (July–September): 99–116.

Bunker, John P. 1970. "Surgical Manpower," *New England Journal of Medicine* 282 (January 15): 135–44.

Burns, Tom, and G. M. Stalker. 1961. *The Management of Innovation* (London: Tavistock).

Burrow, James G. 1963. *AMA, Voice of American Medicine* (Baltimore: Johns Hopkins University Press).

Burrow, James G. 1977. *Organized Medicine in the Progressive Era: The Move toward Monopoly* (Baltimore: Johns Hopkins University Press).

Cameron, Stewart. 1981. *Kidney Diseases: The Facts* (London: Oxford University Press).

Campbell, Donald T., and Julian C. Stanley. 1963. *Experimental and Quasi-Experimental Designs for Research* (Chicago: Rand McNally).

Carder, Mack, and Bendix Klineberg. 1980. "Towards a Salaried Medical Profession: How 'Swedish' was the Seven Crowns Reform?" in Arnold J. Heidenheimer and Nils Elvander, eds., *The Shaping of the Swedish Health System* (New York: St. Martin's Press), 119–42.

Carnoy, Martin. 1984. *The State and Political Theory* (Princeton: Princeton University Press).

Chandler, Alfred D., Jr. 1966. *Strategy and Structure* (New York: Doubleday).

Chandler, Alfred D., Jr. 1977. *The Visible Hand: The Managerial Revolution* (Cambridge: Harvard University Press).

Chen, Milton M., and Douglas P. Wagner. 1978. "Gains in Mortality from Bio-medical Research, 1930–1975: An Initial Assessment," *Social Science and Medicine* 12c: 73– 81.

Cherry, S. 1972. "The Role of the Provincial Hospital: The Norfolk and Norwich Hospital, 1771–1880," *Population Studies* 26: 291–306.

Cherry, S. 1980. "The Hospital and Population Growth: The Voluntary General Hospitals, Mortality, and Local Populations in English Provinces in the Eighteenth and Nineteenth Centuries," *Population Studies* 34: 59–75, 251–65.

Christianson, R. E., et al. 1981. "Incidence of Congenital Anomalies among White and Black Live Births with Long-term Follow-up," *American Journal of Public Health* 71: 1333–41.

Coale, Ansley J., and Melvin Zelnick. 1963. *New Estimates of Fertility and Population in the United States* (Princeton: Princeton University Press).

Cochrane, A. L., A. S. St. Leger, and F. Moore. 1978. "Health Service 'Input' and Mortality 'Output' in Developed Countries," *Journal of Epidemiology and Community Health* 32 (September): 200–5.

Coleman, James S. 1968. "The Concept of Equality of Educational Opportunity," *Harvard Educational Review* 38 (Winter): 7–22.

Coleman, James S. 1973. "Equality of Opportunity and Equality of Results," *Harvard Educational Review* 43 (February): 129–37.

Coleman, James S., et al. 1966. *Equality of Educational Opportunity* (Washington: U.S. Department of Health, Education, and Welfare).

Collins, James J. 1982. "The Contribution of Medical Measures to the Decline of Mortality from Respiratory Tuberculosis: An Age-Period-Cohort Model," *Demography* 19: 409–27.

Collins, Randall. 1974. "Where Are Educational Requirements for Employment Highest?" *Sociology of Education* 47: 419–22.

Collins, Randall. 1979. *The Credential Society* (New York: Academic Press).

Columbia University School of Public Health and Administrative Medicine. 1962. *The Quantity, Quality, and Costs of Medical and Hospital Care Secured by a Sample of Teamster Families in the New York Area* (New York: Teamsters Joint Council no. 16).

Condran, Gretchen A., and Rose A. Cheney. 1982. "Mortality Trends in Philadelphia: Age-and-Cause Specific Death Rates, 1870–1930," *Demography* 19 (February): 97–123.

Condran, Gretchen A., and Eileen Crimmins-Gardner. 1978. "Public Health Measures and Mortality in U.S. Cities in the Late Nineteenth Century," *Human Ecology* 6 (March): 27–54.

Cooper, Michael H. 1974. "Economics of Need: The Experience of the British Health Service," in Mark Perlman, ed., *The Economics of Health and Medical Care* (New York: John Wiley), 89–107.

Cooper, R., et al. 1978. "The Decline in Mortality from Coronary Heart Disease, USA, 1968–1975," *Journal of Chronic Disease* 31: 709–20.

Cooper, Richard, Michael Steinhauer, Arthur Schatzkin, and William Miller. 1981. "Improved Mortality among U.S. Blacks, 1968–1978: The Role of Antiracist Struggle," *International Journal of Health Services* 11: 511–22.

Cornillot, Pierre, and Pierre Bonamour. 1973. "France," in I. Douglas-Wilson and Gordon McLachlan, eds., *Health Services Prospects: An International Survey* (Boston: Little, Brown).

Corwin, Ronald. 1969. "Patterns of Organizational Conflict," *Administrative Science Quarterly* 14 (December): 507–21.

Couder, Brigitte, Georges Rösch, and Simone Sandier. 1972. "La consommation de services médicaux continuera a croître rapidement," *Economie et Statistique* (September): 3–19.

Crane, Diana. 1972. *Invisible Colleges: Diffusion of Knowledge in Scientific Communities* (Chicago: University of Chicago Press).

Crawford, Robert. 1980. "Healthism and the Medicalization of Everyday Life," *International Journal of Health Services* 10: 365–88.

Crimmins, Eileen M. 1981. "The Changing Pattern of American Mortality Decline,

1940–77, and Its Implications for the Future," *Population and Development Review* 7: 229–54.

Crimmins, Eileen M. 1986. "The Social Impact of Recent and Prospective Mortality Declines among Older Americans," *Social Science Research* 70 (April): 192–99.

Culyer, A. J., and B. Harisberger, eds. 1983. *Economic and Medical Evaluation of Health Care Technologies* (Berlin: Springer).

Cuthbert, M. F. 1976. "Developments in the United Kingdom Drug Regulatory System," in P. E. Lucchelli, N. Benjamin, and V. Bachini, eds., *Rationality of Drug Development* (New York: American Elsevier), 81–83.

Dahl, Robert A., and Edward R. Tufte. 1973. *Size and Democracy* (Stanford: Stanford University Press).

Dahlgren, Goran, and Finn Diderichsen. 1986. "Strategies for Equity in Health: Report from Sweden," *International Journal of Health Services* 16: 517–37.

DaSilva, J. C. A. 1975. *The Analysis of Cross-Sectional and Time-Series Data* (Raleigh: Institute of Statistics, North Carolina State University).

Dauer, C. C. 1940. "Smallpox in the United States: Its Decline and Geographic Distribution," *Public Health Reports* 55 (December 13): 2303–12.

David, P. A., and P. Solar. 1977. "A Bicentenary Contribution to the History of the Cost of Living in America," *Research in Economic History* 2: 1–80.

Davis, James E., and Don E. Detmer. 1972. "The Ambulatory Surgical Unit," *Annals of Surgery* 175 (June): 856–62.

Davis, Karen. 1972. "Economic Theories of Behavior in Nonprofit Private Hospitals," *Economic Theories of Behavior* 24 (Winter): 1–13.

Davis, Karen. 1973. "Theories of Hospital Inflation: Some Empirical Evidence," *Journal of Human Resources* 8 (Spring): 181–201.

Davis, Karen. 1975. "Equal Treatment and Unequal Benefits: The Medicare Program," *Milbank Memorial Fund Quarterly* 53 (Fall): 449–88.

Davis, Karen. 1976a. "Achievements and Problems of Medicaid," *Public Health Reports* 91 (July–August): 313–16.

Davis, Karen. 1976b. "Medicaid Payments and Utilization of Medical Services by the Poor," *Inquiry* 13 (June): 122–35.

Davis, Karen. 1977a. "A Decade of Policy Developments in Providing Health Care for Low-Income Families," in Robert Haveman, ed., *A Decade of Federal Antipoverty Programs: Achievements, Failures, and Lessons* (New York: Academic Press), 197–231.

Davis, Karen. 1977b. "Health and the Great Society: Successes of the Past Decade and the Road Ahead," in D. Warner, ed., *Towards New Human Rights: The Social Policies of the Kennedy and Johnson Administrations* (Austin: University of Texas Press).

Davis, Karen, Marsha Gold, and Diane Makuc. 1981. "Access to Health Care for the Poor: Does the Gap Remain?" *Annual Review of Public Health* 2: 159–82.

Davis, Karen, and Diane Rowland. 1983. "Uninsured and Underserved: Inequities in Health Care in the United States," *Milbank Memorial Fund Quarterly* 61 (Spring): 149–76.

Davis, Karen, and Cathy Schoen. 1978. *Health and the War on Poverty: A Ten-Year Appraisal* (Washington, D.C.: Brookings Institution).

Denison, E. F. 1962. *The Sources of Economic Growth in the United States* (New York: Committee for Economic Development).

Denison, E. F. 1967. *Why Growth Rates Differ: Postwar Experience in Nine Western Countries* (Washington, D.C.: Brookings Institution).

Denison, E. F. 1974. *Accounting for United States Economic Growth* (Washington, D.C.: Brookings Institution).

DiMaggio, Paul L., and Walter W. Powell. 1983. "The Iron Cage Revisited: Institutional Isomorphism and Collective Rationality in Organizational Fields," *American Sociological Review* 48 (April): 147–60.

Dixon, C. W. 1962. *Smallpox* (London: J. and A. Churchill).

Donabedian, Avedis. 1976. *Benefits in Medical Care Programs* (Cambridge: Harvard University Press).

Downs, George W. 1976. *Bureaucracy, Innovation, and Public Policy* (Lexington, Mass.: D. C. Heath).

Drummond, Douglas J., and A. Ronald Gallant. 1979. "TSCSREG: A SAS Procedure for the Analysis of Time-Series Cross-Section Data," *SAS Technical Report S-106* (Raleigh, N.C.: SAS Institute).

Duncan, Otis Dudley. 1975. *Introduction to Structural Equation Models* (New York: Academic Press).

Dunlop, Derrick. 1973. "The British System of Drug Regulation," in Richard L. Landon, ed., *Regulating New Drugs* (Chicago: University of Chicago Press), 229–37.

Dupeyroux, Jean-Jacques. 1971. *Sécurité sociale*, 4th ed. (Paris: Palloz).

Durkheim, Emile. 1933. *The Division of Labor in Society* (New York: Macmillan).

Dyhouse, C. 1978. "Working-Class Mothers and Infant Mortality in England, 1895–1914," *Journal of Social History* 12: 248–67.

Easterlin, Richard A. 1977. "Population Issues in American Economic History: A Survey and Critique," in R. E. Gallman, ed., *Recent Developments in the Study of Business and Economic History: Essays in Memory of Herman E. Drooss* (Greenwich, Conn.: Jai Press).

Easterlin, Richard A. 1980. *Birth and Fortune* (New York: Basic Books).

Eckstein, Harry. 1958. *The English Health Service: Its Origins, Structure, and Achievements* (Cambridge: Harvard University Press).

Economic Models. 1976. *The French Health Care System* (Chicago: American Medical Association).

Edmondson, Munro S. 1961. "Neolithic Diffusion Rates," *Current Anthropology* 2 (April): 71–102.

Edwardes, Edmond J. 1903. *A Concise History of Smallpox Vaccination in Europe* (London: H. K. Lewis).

Eggers, Paul W. 1988. "Effects of Transplantation on the Medicare End-Stage Renal Disease Program," *New England Journal of Medicine* 318: 223–29.

Elveback, L. R., D. C. Conolly, and L. T. Kurland. 1981. "Coronary Heart Disease in Residents of Rochester, Minnesota, II: Mortality, Incidence, and Survivorship, 1950–1975," *Mayo Clinic Proceedings* 56: 665–72.

Enthoven, Alain C. 1978. "Shattuck Lecture: Cutting the Cost without Cutting the Quality of Care," *New England Journal of Medicine* 298 (June 1): 1229–38.

Enthoven, Alain C. 1980. *Health Plan: The Only Practical Solution to the Soaring Cost of Medical Care* (Reading, Mass.: Addison-Wesley).

Enthoven, Alain C. 1981. "The Behavior of Health Care Agents: Provider Behavior," in Jacques Van Der Gaag and Mark Perlman, eds., *Health, Economics, and Health Economics* (Amsterdam: North-Holland).

Erhardt, Carl L., et al. 1970. "An Epidemiological Approach to Infant Mortality," *Archives of Environmental Health* 20 (June): 743–57.

Erhardt, Carl L., and J. E. Berlin, eds. 1974. *Mortality and Morbidity in the United States* (Cambridge: Harvard University Press).

Evans, Peter B., Dietrich Rueschemeyer, and Theda Skocpol, eds. 1985. *Bringing the State Back In* (Cambridge: Cambridge University Press).

Evans, Robert G. 1974. "Supplier-Induced Demand: Some Empirical Evidence and Implications," in Mark Perlman, ed., *The Economics of Health and Medical Care* (New York: John Wiley), 162–73.

Evans, Robert G. 1981. "Incomplete Vertical Integration: The Distinctive Structure of the Care Industry," in J. Van Der Gaag and M. Perlman, eds., *Health, Economics, and Health Economics* (Amsterdam: North-Holland), 329–54.

Evans, R. W. et al. 1981. "A Social and Demographic Profile of Hemodialysis Patients in the United States," *Journal of the American Medical Association* 245: 487–91.

Eveleth, P. B., and J. M. Tanner. 1976. *Worldwide Variation in Human Growth* (Cambridge: Cambridge University Press).

Eyler, John M. 1979. *Victorian Social Medicine* (Baltimore: Johns Hopkins University Press).

Falk, I. S., et al. 1933. *The Incidence of Illness and the Receipt and Costs of Medical Care among Representative Families* (Chicago: University of Chicago Press).

Farkas, Suzanne. 1971. "The Federal Role in Urban Decentralization," *American Behavioral Scientist* 15 (September–October): 15–35.

Fein, Rashi. 1967. *The Doctor Shortage: An Economic Diagnosis* (Washington, D.C.: Brookings Institution).

Feldstein, Martin S. 1967. *Economic Analysis for Health Service Efficiency* (Amsterdam: North-Holland).

Feldstein, Martin S. 1970. "The Rising Price of Physician's Services," *Review of Economics and Statistics* 52 (May): 121–33.

Feldstein, Martin S. 1973. "The Welfare Loss of Excess Health Insurance," *Journal of Political Economy* 81 (March/April): 251–80.

Feldstein, Martin S., and Bernard Friedman. 1977. "Tax Subsidies, the Rational Demand for Insurance, and the Health Care Crisis," *Journal of Public Economics* 7: 155–78.

Fesler, James W. 1965. "Approaches to the Understanding of Decentralization," *Journal of Politics* 27 (August): 537–66.

Fingerhut, L. A., R. W. Wilson, and J. J. Feldman. 1980. "Health and Disease in the United States," *Annual Review of Public Health* 1: 1–36.

Fitzhardinge, P. W., and E. M. Steven. 1972. "The Small-for-Date Infant, I: Later Growth Patterns," *Pediatrics* 49: 671–81.

Fliegel, F. C., J. E. Kivlin, and G. S. Sekhon. 1968. "A Cross-Cultural Comparison of Farmer's Perception of Innovations as Related to Adoption Behavior," *Rural Sociology* 33 (December): 437–49.

Flinn, M. W. 1982. "The Population History of England, 1541–1871," *Economic History Review* 35: 443–57.

Flora, Peter. 1983. *State, Economy, and Society in Western Europe, 1815–1975* (Chicago: St. James Press).

Flora, Peter, and Arnold Heidenheimer, eds. 1981. *The Development of Welfare States in Europe and America* (New Brunswick, N.J.: Transaction Books).

Floud, R. 1983a. "Inference from the Heights of Volunteer Soldiers and Sailors," National Bureau of Economic Research, mimeo.

Floud, R. 1983b. "The Heights of Europeans since 1750: A New Source for European Economic History," Birkbeck College, London, mimeo.

Floud, R., and K. W. Wachter. 1982. "Poverty and Physical Stature: Evidence on the Standard of Living of London Boys, 1770–1870," *Social Science History* 6: 422–52.

Floud, R., and K. W. Wachter. 1983. "The Physical State of the British Working Class, 1860–1914: Evidence from Army Recruits," Birkbeck College, London, mimeo.

Fogel, Robert W. 1986. "Nutrition and the Decline of Mortality since 1700: Some Additional Preliminary Findings," National Bureau of Economic Research Working Paper no. 1802.

Forbes, Duncan. 1937. "Vaccinations in the Control of Smallpox," *Lancet* (January 16): 174–75.

Forbes, William H. 1967. "Longevity and Medical Costs," *New England Journal of Medicine* 227 (July 13): 71–78.

Forsdahl, A. 1977. "Are Poor Living Conditions in Childhood and Adolescence an Important Risk Factor for Arteriosclerotic Heart Disease?" *British Journal of Preventive and Social Medicine* 31: 91–95.

Foucault, Michel. 1963. *Naissance de la clinique: Une archéologie du regard médical* (Paris: Presses Universitaires Françaises).

Fowler, William. 1927. "Smallpox Vaccination Laws, Regulations, and Court Decisions," *Public Health Reports*, Supplement no. 60 (Washington, D.C.: GPO), 1–74.

Fox, Daniel M. 1986. "The Consequences of Consensus: American Health Policy in the Twentieth Century," *Milbank Quarterly*, 64.1: 76–99.

Freeman, Christopher, ed. 1986. *Design, Innovation, and Long Cycles in Economic Development* (New York: St. Martin's Press).

Freymann, John G. 1974. *The American Health Care System: Its Genesis and Trajectory* (New York: Medcom Press).

Friedman, Milton. 1955. "The Role of Government in Education," in *Economics and the Public Interest* (New Brunswick: Rutgers University Press).

Friedman, Milton, and Simon Kuznets. 1945. *Income from Independent Professional Practice* (New York: National Bureau of Economic Research).

Fries, J. F. 1980. "Aging, Natural Death, and the Compression of Morbidity," *New England Journal of Medicine* 303 (July 17): 130–35.

Fries, J. F. 1983. "The Compression of Morbidity," *Milbank Memorial Fund Quarterly* 61 (Summer): 397–419.

Fries, J. F., and L. M. Crapo. 1981. *Vitality and Aging: Implications of the Rectangular Curve* (San Francisco: W. H. Freeman, 1981).

Frisancho, A. R. 1978. "Nutritional Influences on Human Growth and Maturation," *Yearbook of Physical Anthropology* 21: 174–91.

Fry, John, and W. John Stephen. 1986. "Primary Health Care in the United Kingdom," *International Journal of Health Services* 16: 485–96.

Fuchs, Victor R. 1974a. "Some Economic Aspects of Mortality in Developed Countries," in Mark Perlman, ed., *The Economics of Health and Medical Care* (New York: John Wiley), 174–93.

Fuchs, Victor R. 1974b. *Who Shall Live?* (New York: Basic Books).

Fuchs, Victor R. 1986. *The Health Economy* (Cambridge: Harvard University Press).

Fuchs, Victor R., and M. J. Kramer. 1972. *Determinants of Expenditures for Physicians'*

Services in the United States. 1948–1968 (New York: National Bureau of Economic Research, Occasional Paper no. 117).

Garnier, Maurice, and Michael Hout. 1981. "Schooling Processes and Educational Outcomes in France," *Quality and Quantity* 15: 151–77.

Gibson, Robert. 1980. "National Health Care Expenditures, 1979," *Health Care Financing Review* (Summer): 17–29.

Gilbert, Bentley B. 1966. *The Evolution of National Insurance in Great Britain* (London: Joseph).

Gilbert, Bentley B. 1970. *British Social Policy, 1914–1939* (Ithaca: Cornell University Press).

Gillum, R. F., A. R. Folsom, and H. Blackburn. 1984. "Decline in Coronary Heart Disease Mortality: Old Questions and New Facts," *American Journal of Medicine* 76: 1055–65.

Glaser, William A. 1970. *Paying the Doctor* (Baltimore: Johns Hopkins University Press).

Glaser, William A. 1983. "Paying the Hospital: Foreign Lessons for the United States," *Health Care Financing Review* 4 (Summer): 99–110.

Glass, Gene V., Victor L. Willson, and John M. Gottman. 1975. *Design and Analysis of Time-Series Experiments* (Boulder: Colorado Associated University Press).

Goldman, L., and F. Cook, et al. 1984. "The Decline in Ischemic Heart Disease Mortality Rates," *Annals of Internal Medicine* 101: 825–36.

Goldsmith, Jeff Charles. 1981. *Can Hospitals Survive? The New Competitive Health Care Market* (Homewood, Ill.: Dow Jones-Irwin).

Goldthorpe, John H., ed. 1984. *Order and Conflict in Contemporary Capitalism: Studies in the Political Economy of Western European Nations* (Oxford: Oxford University Press).

Gortmaker, Steven L. 1979. "Poverty and Infant Mortality in the United States," *American Sociological Review* 44: 280–97.

Grabowski, Henry G. 1976. *Drug Regulation and Innovation: Empirical Evidence and Policy Options* (Washington, D.C.: American Enterprise Institute).

Graham-Smith, D. G. 1981. "Problems Facing a Regulatory Authority," in J. F. Cavalla, ed., *Risk-Benefit Analysis in Drug Research* (Lancaster: MTP Press), 51–61.

Gray, Virginia. 1973. "Innovation in the States: A Diffusion Study," *American Political Science Review* 67 (December): 1174–85.

Great Britain, House of Commons. 1889, 1896, 1897. *Royal Commission on Vaccination* (cmd. 5845, 8270, 7993).

Great Britain, House of Commons. 1890. *The Royal Commission on Vaccinations*, vol. 39.

Great Britain, House of Commons. 1904. *Report of the Interdepartmental Committee on Physical Deterioration*, vol. 1.

Great Britain, House of Commons. 1910. *Epidemic Diseases in England and Wales* (cmd. 5312).

Great Britain, Ministry of Health. 1931. "A Review of Certain Present Aspects of Smallpox Prevention," *Reports on Public Health and Medical Subjects*, no. 62 (London: HMSO).

Great Britain, Office of Population Censuses and Surveys. 1891–1983. *Decennial Census* (London: HMSO).

Great Britain, Registrar General. 1891–1971. Reports (London: HMSO).

Grew, Raymond, ed. 1978. *Crises of Political Development in Europe and the United States* (Princeton: Princeton University Press).

Griliches, Zvi. 1957. "Hybrid Corn: An Exploration in the Economics of Technological Change," *Econometrica* 25 (October): 501–22.

Grossman, Michael. 1972. *The Demand for Health: A Theoretical and Empirical Investigation* (New York: Columbia University Press).

Grossman, Michael. 1976. "The Correlation between Health and Schooling," in Nestor E. Terleckyj, ed., *Household Production and Consumption* (New York: Columbia University Press), 147–211.

Grossman, Michael, and Steven Jacobowitz. 1981. "Variations in Infant Mortality Rates among Counties of the United States: The Roles of Public Policies and Programs," *Demography* 18 (November): 695–713.

Grove, Robert D., and Alice M. Hetzel. 1968. *Vital Statistics Rates in the United States, 1940–1960* (Washington, D.C.: National Center for Health Statistics).

Guinchard, J. 1914. *Sweden: Historical and Statistical Handbook* (Stockholm: Norstedt).

Guralnick, Lillian. 1963. *Mortality by Occupation and Cause of Death among Men 20 to 64 Years of Age: United States, 1950*, Vital Statistics Special Reports no. 53 (Washington, D.C.: GPO).

Habakkuk, H. J. 1971. *Population Growth and Economic Development since 1750* (Leicester: Leicester University Press).

Habicht, J. P., C. Yarbrough, and R. Martorelli. 1979. "Anthropometric Field Methods: Criteria for Selection," in D. B. Jelliffe and E. F. P. Jelliffe, eds., *Nutrition and Growth* (New York: Plenum Press), 365–87.

Hadley, Jack. 1982. *More Medical Care, Better Health?* (Washington, D.C.: Urban Institute).

Hage, Jerald. 1965. "An Axiomatic Theory of Organizations," *Administrative Science Quarterly* 10 (December): 289–320.

Hage, Jerald. 1972. *Techniques and Problems of Theory Construction in Sociology* (New York: Wiley-Interscience).

Hage, Jerald. 1974. *Communication and Organization Control* (New York: John Wiley).

Hage, Jerald. 1980. *Theories of Organizations: Form, Process, and Transformation* (New York: John Wiley).

Hage, Jerald, and Michael Aiken. 1967. "Program Change and Organizational Properties: A Comparative Analysis," *American Journal of Sociology* 72 (March): 503–19.

Hage, Jerald, and Michael Aiken. 1969. "Routine Technology, Social Structure, and Organizational Goals," *Administrative Science Quarterly* 14 (September): 366–77.

Hage, Jerald, and Michael Aiken. 1970. *Social Change in Complex Organizations* (New York: Random House).

Hage, Jerald, and Robert Dewar. 1973. "Elite Values versus Organizational Structure in Predicting Innovation," *Administrative Science Quarterly* 18 (September): 279–90.

Hage, Jerald, Robert Hanneman, and Edward T. Gargan. 1989. *State Responsiveness and State Activism: An Examination of the Social Forces and State Strategies That Explain the Rise in Social Expenditures in Britain, France, Germany, and Italy, 1870–1968* (London: Unwin Hyman).

Hage, Jerald, and J. Rogers Hollingsworth. 1977. "The First Steps toward the Integration of Social Theory and Social Policy," *Annals of the American Academy of Political and Social Science* 434 (November): 1–23.

Hage, Jerald, J. Rogers Hollingsworth, and Robert Hanneman. 1981. "Social Efficiency of Health Care Systems: A Longitudinal Analysis of Britain, France,

Sweden, and the United States," *Scandinavian Journal of Social Medicine* Supplement, 28: 9–44.

Haider, Donald. 1971. "The Political Economy of Decentralization," *American Behavioral Scientist* 15 (September–October): 108–29.

Haines, Blanche M. 1930. "Effect of Antepartum Care of the Mother," *American Journal of Public Health* 20 (March): 273–76.

Haines, Michael R. 1983. "Differential Child Mortality by Occupation and Social Class of Parents: Evidence from the United States, 1900, and England and Wales, 1911," Paper presented to the Population Association of America, Pittsburgh, Pennsylvania, April 14–16.

Hall, Peter. 1983. "Policy Innovation and the Structure of the State: The Politics-Administration Nexus in France and Britain," *Annals of the American Academy of Political and Social Sciences* 466: 43–59.

Hall, Richard H. 1977. *Organization Structure and Process*, 2d ed. (Englewood Cliffs, N.J.: Prentice-Hall).

Halls, W. D. 1965. *Society, Schools, and Progress in France* (London: Pergamon Press).

Ham, Christopher. 1988. "Governing the Health Sector: Power and Policy Making in the English and Swedish Health Services," *Milbank Quarterly* 66.2: 389–414.

Hamblin, Robert L., R. Brooke Jacobsen, and Jerry L. L. Miller. 1973. *A Mathematical Theory of Social Change* (New York: John Wiley).

Hanneman, Robert, and J. Rogers Hollingsworth. 1984. "Modeling and Simulation in Historical Inquiry," *Historical Methods* 17 (Summer): pts. 1 and 2, 150–63.

Hardy, Anne. 1988. "Diagnosis, Death, and Diet: The Case of London, 1750–1909," *Journal of Interdisciplinary History* 18: 387–402.

Hardyment, Christina. 1983. *Dream Babies* (London: Jonathan Cape).

Hatzfeld, Henri. 1963. *Le grand tournant de la médecine libérale* (Paris: Economie et Humanisme).

Hatzfeld, Henri. 1971. *Du pauperisme à la sécurité sociale: Essai sur les origines de la sécurité sociale en France, 1850–1940* (Paris: Armand Colin).

Haveman, Robert H., et al. 1974. *Benefit-Cost and Policy Analysis* (Chicago: Aldine).

Hayflick, L. 1965. "The Limited *in Vitro* Lifetime of Human Diploid Cell Strains," *Experimental Cell Research* 37: 614–36.

Hayflick, L. 1975. "Current Theories of Biological Aging," *Federation Proceedings of American Societies for Experimental Biology* 34: 9–13.

Hayflick, L. 1977. "Perspectives on Human Longevity," in B. Neugarten and R. Havighurst, eds., *Extending the Human Life Span: Social Policy and Social Ethics* (Chicago: Committee on Human Development, University of Chicago), 1–12.

Heckscher, Eli F. 1954. *An Economic History of Sweden* (Cambridge: Harvard University Press).

Heclo, Hugh. 1974. *Modern Social Politics in Britain and Sweden* (New Haven: Yale University Press).

Heidenheimer, Arnold J. 1980. "Conflict and Compromises between Professional and Bureaucratic Health Interests, 1947–1972," in Heidenheimer and Nils Elvander, eds., *The Shaping of the Swedish Health System* (New York: St. Martin's Press), 119–42.

Heidenheimer, Arnold, and Nils Elvander, eds. 1980. *The Shaping of the Swedish Health System* (New York: St. Martin's Press).

Held, Phillip J., et al. 1988. "Access to Kidney Transplantation: Has the United

States Eliminated Income and Racial Differences?" *Archives of Internal Medicine* 148: 2594–2600.

Herlitz, Nils. 1939. *Sweden: A Modern Democracy on Ancient Foundations* (Minneapolis: University of Minnesota Press).

Hessler, Richard M., and Andrew C. Twaddle. 1982. "Sweden's Crisis in Medical Care: Political and Legal Changes," *Journal of Health Politics, Policy, and Law* 7 (Summer): 440–59.

Higgs, Robert. 1971. *The Transformation of the American Economy, 1865–1914* (New York: John Wiley).

Higgs, Robert. 1979. "Cycles and Trends of Mortality in 18 Large American Cities, 1871–1900," *Explorations in Entrepreneurial History* 16: 381–408.

Hoeprich, Paul D. 1976. *Infectious Diseases: A Modern Treatise of Infectious Processes* (New York: Harper and Row).

Hogarth, James. 1963. *The Payment of the General Practitioner* (New York: Pergamon Press).

Hollingsworth, J. Rogers. 1971. "An Approach to the Study of Comparative Historical Politics," in Hollingsworth, ed., *Nation and State Building in America: Comparative Historical Perspectives* (Boston: Little, Brown), 251–77.

Hollingsworth, J. Rogers. 1974. "Problems of Theory Construction in Historical Analysis," *Historical Methods* 7 (June): 225–44.

Hollingsworth, J. Rogers. 1979. "Inequality in Levels of Health in England and Wales, 1891–1971." Institute for Research on Poverty, University of Wisconsin, Discussion Paper no. 578–79.

Hollingsworth, J. Rogers. 1981. "Inequality in Levels of Health in England and Wales," *Journal of Health and Social Behavior* 22 (September): 268–83.

Hollingsworth, J. Rogers. 1982. "The Political-Structural Basis for Economic Performance," *Annals of the American Academy of Political and Social Science* 459 (January): 28–45.

Hollingsworth, J. Rogers. 1983. "Causes and Consequences of the American Medical System," *Reviews in American History* 11 (September): 326–32.

Hollingsworth, J. Rogers. 1984. "The Snare of Specialization," *Bulletin of Atomic Scientists* 40 (June): 34–37.

Hollingsworth, J. Rogers. 1986. *A Political Economy of Medicine: Great Britain and the United States* (Baltimore: John Hopkins University Press).

Hollingsworth, J. Rogers, Jerald Hage, and Robert Hanneman. 1978. "The Impact of the Organization of Health Delivery Systems on Health Efficiency: A Comparative Analysis of the United States, France, and Great Britain," Paper for the American Sociological Association, San Francisco, September 4.

Hollingsworth, J. Rogers, and Robert Hanneman. 1982. "Working-Class Power and the Political Economy of Western Capitalist Societies," *Comparative Social Research* 5: 61–80.

Hollingsworth, J. Rogers, and Robert Hanneman. 1984. *Centralization and Power in Social Service Delivery Systems* (Boston: Kluwer Nijhoff).

Hollingsworth, J. Rogers, and Ellen Jane Hollingsworth. 1985. "Differences between Voluntary and Public Organizations: The Behavior of Hospitals in England and Wales," *Journal of Health Politics, Policy, and Law* 10 (Summer): 371–97.

Hollingsworth, J. Rogers, and Ellen Jane Hollingsworth. 1987. *Controversy about American Hospitals: Funding, Ownership, and Performance* (Washington, D.C.: American Enterprise Institute).

Hollingsworth, J. Rogers, and Leon N. Lindberg. 1985. "The Governance of the American Economy: The Role of Markets, Clans, Hierarchies, and Associative Behaviour," in Wolfgang Streeck and Philippe C. Schmitter, eds., *Private Interest Government* (Beverly Hills, Calif.: Sage), 221–54.

Husen, Torsten. 1969a. "Responsiveness and Resistance in the Educational System to Changing Needs of Society: Some Swedish Experiences," *International Review of Education* 15: 476–85.

Husen, Torsten. 1969b. *Talent, Opportunity, and Career: A Twenty-Six Year Follow-up of 1,500 Individuals* (Stockholm: Almquist and Wiksell).

Illich, Ivan. 1976. *Medical Nemesis: The Expropriation of Health* (New York: Pantheon).

Imbert, Jean. 1972. "Dossiers themis," *L'hôpital français* (Paris: Presses Universitaires Françaises).

Institut National de la Statistique et des Études Économiques pour la Metropole et la France d'Outre-Mer. Various years. *Annuaire statistique de la France.*

International Labor Office, 1959. *The Cost of Medical Care* (Geneva: ILO).

Ito, Hirobumi. 1980. "Health Insurance and Medical Services in Sweden and Denmark, 1850–1950," in Arnold J. Heidenheimer and Nils Elvander, eds., *The Shaping of the Swedish Health System* (New York: St. Martin's Press), 44–67.

Jacobs, Philip. 1974. "A Survey of Economic Models of Hospitals," *Inquiry* 10 (June): 83–97.

Jencks, Christopher, et al. 1972. *Inequality: A Reassessment of the Effect of Family and Schooling in America* (New York: Basic Books).

Johnston, Robert F., and Kenneth H. Wildrick. 1974. "'State of the Art': Review of the Impact of Chemotherapy on the Care of Patients with Tuberculosis," *American Review of Respiratory Disease* 109: 636–64.

Jolly, Dominique. 1973. "La formation médicale continue et la rentabilité de l'investissement humain chez les praticiens" (Thèse pour le doctorat, Université de Paris I).

Jonsson, Bengt. 1981. *The Costs of Health Care: Trends and Determining Factors* (Lund, Sweden: Institutet for Halso-Och Sjukvardsekonomi).

Joskow, Paul. 1980. "Alternative Regulatory Mechanisms for Controlling Hospital Costs" (Paper presented before the Conference on Health Care: Professional Ethics, Government Regulation, or Markets? September 25–26).

Kaluzny, Arnold D., James E. Veney, and John T. Gentry. 1974. "Innovation of Health Services: A Comparative Study of Hospitals and Health Departments," *Milbank Memorial Fund Quarterly* 52 (Winter): 51–82.

Karpik, Lucien. 1972a. "Le capitalisme technologique," *Sociologie du Travail* 13 (January–March): 2–34.

Karpik, Lucien. 1972b. "Les politiques et les logics d'action de la grande entreprise industrielle," *Sociologie du Travail* 13 (April–June): 82–105.

Katz, Elihu, Herbert Hamilton, and Marvin Levin. 1963. "Traditions of Research on the Diffusion of Innovation," *American Sociological Review* 28 (April): 237–52.

Katzenstein, Peter. 1984. *Corporatism and Change: Austria, Switzerland, and the Politics of Industry* (Ithaca: Cornell University Press).

Katzenstein, Peter. 1985. *Small States in World Markets: Industrial Policy in Europe* (Ithaca: Cornell University Press).

Kenny, David A. 1979. *Correlation and Causality* (New York: John Wiley).

Kerr, J. W. 1912. "Vaccination: An Analysis of the Laws and Regulations Relating Thereto in Force in the United States," *Public Health Bulletin*, no. 52 (Washington, D.C.: GPO).

Kessner, David M., et al. 1973. *Infant Death: An Analysis by Maternal Risk and Health Care*, vol. 1 (Washington, D.C.: National Academy of Sciences).

Keyfitz, N. 1978. "Improving Life Expectancy: An Uphill Road Ahead," *American Journal of Public Health* 68: 954–56.

Keyfitz, N., and W. Flieger. 1971. *Population: Facts and Methods of Demography* (San Francisco: W. H. Freeman).

Kielmann, A. A., et al. 1983. *Child and Maternal Health Services in Rural India: The Narangival Experiment*, vol. 1: *Integrated Nutrition and Health* (Baltimore: Johns Hopkins University Press).

Kinzer, David. 1988. "The Decline and Fall of Deregulation," *New England Journal of Medicine* 318 (January 14): 112–16.

Kitagawa, Evelyn, and Philip M. Hauser. 1973. *Differential Mortality in the United States* (Cambridge: Harvard University Press).

Klein, Rudolf. 1983. *The Politics of the National Health Service* (London: Longman).

Kleinman, Joel C. 1986. "State Trends in Infant Mortality, 1968–83," *American Journal of Public Health* 76 (June): 681–86.

Kmenta, Jan. 1986. *Elements of Econometrics*, 2d ed. (New York: Macmillan).

Kolata, Gina. 1981. "Consensus on CT Scans," *Science* 214 (December 18): 1327–28.

Kolata, Gina. 1983. "Some Bypass Surgery Unnecessary," *Science* 222 (November 11): 605.

Komlos, John. 1985. "Stature and Nutrition in the Habsburg Monarchy: The Standard of Living and Economic Development in the Eighteenth Century," *American Historical Review* 90: 1149–61.

Komlos, John. 1986. "Patterns of Children's Growth in East-Central Europe in the Eighteenth Century," *Annals of Human Biology* 13: 33–48.

Komlos, John. 1987. "The Height and Weight of West Point Cadets: Dietary Changes in Antebellum America," *Journal of Economic History* 47: 897–928.

Komlos, John. 1988. "The Food Budget of English Workers: A Comment on Shammas," *Journal of Economic History* 48: 149.

Korpi, Walter. 1978. *The Working Class in Welfare Capitalism* (London: Routledge & Kegan Paul).

Korpi, Walter. 1983. *The Democratic Class Struggle* (London: Routledge & Kegan Paul).

Krakauer, H., et al. 1983. "The Recent U.S. Experience in the Treatment of End-Stage Renal Diseases by Dialysis and Transplantation," *New England Journal of Medicine* 308 (June 30): 1558–63.

Kronenfeld, Jennie J., and Marcia Lynn Whicker. 1984. *U.S. National Health Policy* (New York: Praeger).

Krueger, Marlls, and Baerbel Wallisch-Prinz. 1972. "University Reform in Progress: The Current Debate in West Germany," *Comparative Education Review* 16 (June): 340–51.

Kuh, Edwin. 1959. "The Validity of Cross-Sectionally Estimated Behavior Equations in Time-Series Applications," *Econometrica* 27: 197–214.

Kunitz, S. J. 1983. "Speculations on the European Mortality Decline," *Economic History Review* 36: 349–64.

Lambert, R. J. 1962. "A Victorian National Health Service: State Vaccination, 1855–1871," *Historical Journal* 5: 1–18.

Law, Sylvia. 1974. *Blue Cross: What Went Wrong?* (New Haven: Yale University Press).

Lawrence, Paul R., and Jay W. Lorsch. 1967. "Differentiation and Integration in Complex Organizations," *Administrative Science Quarterly* 12 (June): 1–47.

Layet, A. 1886. "Le service municipal de la préservation de la variole a Bordeaux," *Revue d'Hygiene* 8: 759–71.

Leavitt, Judith Walzer. 1982. *The Healthiest City: Milwaukee and the Politics of Health Reform* (Princeton: Princeton University Press).

Lee, Maw Lin. 1971. "A Conspicuous Production Theory of Hospital Behavior," *Southern Economic Journal* 38 (July): 48–58.

Lefcowitz, Myron J. 1973. "Poverty and Health: A Re-examination," *Inquiry* 10 (March): 3–13.

Le Grand, Julian, and Ray Robinson, eds. 1984. *Privatization and the Welfare State* (London: George Allen and Unwin).

Le Roy Ladurie, Emmanuel. 1974. *The Peasants of France*, trans. John Day (Urbana: University of Illinois Press).

Levin, Henry M., ed. 1970. *Community Control of Schools* (Washington, D.C.: Brookings Institution).

Levitt Theodore. 1975. "Marketing Myopia," *Harvard Business Review* 53 (September–October): 26–44, 173–81.

Levy, E., et al. 1982. *La croissance des dépenses de santé* (Paris: Economica).

Levy, Hermann. 1944. *National Health Insurance: A Critical Study* (Cambridge: Cambridge University Press).

Levy, Robert I. 1981. "The Decline in Cardiovascular Disease Mortality," *Annual Review of Public Health* 2: 49–70.

Levy-Lambert, H., and H. Guillaume. 1971. *La rationalisation des choix budgétaires* (Paris: Presses Universitaires Françaises).

Lewis, Charles E. 1969. "Variations in the Incidence of Surgery," *New England Journal of Medicine* 281 (October 16): 880–84.

Lewis, Jane. 1980. "The Social History of Social Policy: Infant Welfare in Edwardian England," *Journal of Social Policy* 9: 463–86.

Lewis, L. 1980. *The Politics of Motherhood: Child and Maternal Welfare in England, 1900–1939* (London: Croom Helm).

Lewis, R. A. 1952. *Edwin Chadwick and the Public Health Movement* (London: Longmans, Green).

Lindblom, Charles. 1959. "The Science of 'Muddling Through,'" *Public Administration Review* 19 (Spring): 79–88.

Lindblom, Charles E. 1977. *Politics and Markets* (New York: Basic Books).

Lindert, P. H. 1983. "English Living Standards, Population Growth, and Wrigley-Schofield," *Explorations in Economic History* 20: 131–55.

Lindert, P. H., and J. G. Williamson. 1983. "English Workers' Living Standards during the Industrial Revolution: A New Look," *Economic History Review* 36: 1–25.

Lindsay, Cotton M. 1978. *The Pharmaceutical Industry: Economic Performance and Government Regulation* (New York: John Wiley).

Lindsay, Cotton M., and A. Seldon. 1980. *National Health Issues: The British Experience* (New York: Roche Laboratories).

Lindsey, Almont. 1962. *Socialized Medicine in England and Wales: The National Health Service, 1948–1961* (Chapel Hill: University of North Carolina Press).

Litman, Theodor J., and Leonard S. Robins, eds. 1984. *Health Politics and Policy* (New York: John Wiley).

Lockhart, Charles. 1984. "Explaining Social Policy Differences among Advanced Industrial Societies," *Comparative Politics* 16 (April): 335–56.

Lodeon, Marie-Christine. 1970. "La rationalisation des choix budgétaires dans le secteur sanitaire," *Analyse et Prévision* 9: 89–100.

4

4

Logan, W. P. D. 1950. "Mortality in England and Wales from 1848 to 1947," *Population Studies* 4 (September): 132–78.

Logan, W. P. D., and Eileen Brooke. 1957. *The Survey of Sickness, 1943–1952*, Studies on Medical and Population Subjects, no. 12 (London: HMSO).

Loschky, David J. 1976. "Economic Change, Mortality, and Malthusian Theory," *Population Studies* 30 (November): 439–52.

Luckin, Bill. 1984. "Evaluating the Sanitary Revolution: Typhus and Typhoid in London, 1851–1900," in Robert Woods and John Woodward, eds., *Urban Disease and Mortality in Nineteenth-Century England* (New York: St. Martin's Press), 102–19.

Luft, Harold S., John Bunker, and Alain C. Enthoven. 1979. "Should Operations Be Regionalized? The Empirical Relation between Surgical Volume and Mortality," *New England Journal of Medicine* 301 (December 20): 1364–69.

McCarthy, Carol M. 1988. "Financing Indigent Care: Short- and Long-term Strategies," *Journal of the American Medical Association* 259: 75.

McCleary, J. F. 1933. *The Early History of the Infant Welfare Movement* (London: H. K. Lewis).

McCormick, M. C. 1985. "The Contribution of Low Birth Weight to Infant Mortality and Childhood Morbidity," *New England Journal of Medicine* 312: 82–89.

McKeown, Thomas. 1975. *Medicine in Modern Society* (London: George Allen and Unwin).

McKeown, Thomas. 1976a. *The Modern Rise of Population* (New York: Academic Press).

McKeown, Thomas. 1976b. *The Role of Medicine: Dream, Mirage, or Nemesis* (London: Nuffield Provincial Hospital Trust).

McKeown, Thomas. 1978. "Fertility, Mortality, and Causes of Death: An Examination of Issues Related to the Modern Rise of Population," *Population Studies* 32 (November): 535–42.

McKeown, Thomas. 1983. "Food, Infection, and Population," *Journal of Interdisciplinary History* 14 (Autumn): 227–47.

McKeown, Thomas, and R. G. Record. 1962. "An Interpretation of the Decline of Mortality in England and Wales during the Nineteenth Century," *Population Studies* 16 (November): 94–122.

McKeown, Thomas, R. G. Record, and R. D. Turner. 1975. "An Interpretation of the Decline of Mortality in England and Wales during the Twentieth Century," *Population Studies* 29 (November): 391–422.

McKinlay, John B. 1979. "Epidemiological and Political Determinants of Social Policies regarding the Public Health," *Social Science and Medicine* 13A: 541–58.

McKinlay, John B., and Sonja M. McKinlay. 1977. "The Questionable Contribution of Medical Measures to the Decline of Mortality in the United States in the Twentieth Century," *Milbank Memorial Fund Quarterly* 55 (Summer): 405–28.

Macleod, Roy M. 1967. "The Frustration of State Medicine, 1880–1889," *Medical History* 11: 15–40.

McNerney, Walter J. 1980. "Control of Health-Care Costs in the 1980s," *New England Journal of Medicine* 303 (November 6): 1088–95.

McPhee, Stephen J., and Steven A. Schroeder, 1987. "Promoting Preventive Care: Changing Reimbursement Is Not Enough," *American Journal of Public Health* 77: 278–81.

MacPherson, Lisa A. 1986. "Coronary Heart Disease and Related Technologies: A Case Study in Technology Assessment." Unpublished paper, University of Wisconsin.

Maddala, G. S. 1971. "The Use of Variance Components Models in Pooling Cross-Section and Time-Series Data," *Econometrica* 39: 341–58.

Maddick, R. 1960. "Some Effects of Technical Innovations on the Relationship between Central and Local Authorities," *International Social Science Journal* 12: 385–93.

Manga, Pranial, and Geoffrey R. Weller. 1980. "The Failure of the Equity Objective in Health: A Comparative Analysis of Canada, Britain, and the United States," *Comparative Social Research* 3: 229–67.

Mansfield, Edwin. 1961. "Technical Change and the Rate of Imitation," *Econometrica* 29 (October): 741–66.

Mansfield, Edwin. 1968a. *The Economics of Technological Change* (New York: Norton).

Mansfield, Edwin. 1968b. *Industrial Research and Technological Innovation: An Econometric Analysis* (New York: Norton).

Manton, Kenneth G. 1982. "Changing Concepts of Morbidity and Mortality in the Elderly Population," *Milbank Memorial Fund Quarterly* 60 (Spring): 183–244.

March, James G., and Herbert A. Simon. 1958. *Organizations* (New York: John Wiley).

Margo, Robert A., and Richard H. Steckel. 1983. "Heights of Native-Born Whites during the Antebellum Period," *Journal of Economic History* 43: 167–74.

Marmor, Theodore R. 1973. *The Politics of Medicine* (Chicago: Aldine).

Marmor, Theodore R. 1977. "The Policies of National Health Insurance: Analysis and Prescription," *Policy Analysis* 3 (Winter): 25–48.

Marmor, Theodore R., and D. Thomas. 1971. "The Politics of Paying Physicians: The Determinants of Government Payment Methods in England, Sweden, and the United States," *International Journal of Health Services* 1: 71–78.

Marmot, M. G., M. J. Shipley, and G. Rose. 1984. "Inequalities in Death-Specific Explanations of a General Pattern," *Lancet* 1 (May 5), 1003–6.

Marx, Karl. 1967. *Essential Writings of Karl Marx*, ed. David Conte (London: MacGibben and Kee).

Marx, Karl, and Friedrich Engels. 1947. *The German Ideology* (New York: International).

Maxwell, Robert J. 1981. *Health and Wealth* (Lexington, Mass.: D. C. Heath).

May, J. M. 1958. *The Ecology of Human Disease* (New York: M.D. Publications).

Mead, Lawrence M. 1977. *Institutional Analysis: An Approach to Implementation Problems in Medicaid* (Washington, D.C.: Urban Institute).

Mechanic, David. 1972. *Public Expectations and Public Health* (New York: John Wiley).

Meeker, Edward. 1972. "The Improving Health of the United States, 1850–1915," *Explorations in Economic History* 9: 353–73.

Meigs, Grace. 1917. *Maternal Mortality from All Conditions in the United States and Certain Other Countries*, Children's Bureau Misc. no. 6, Bureau Publications no. 19 (Washington, D.C.: GPO).

Meijer, Hans. 1969. "Bureaucracy and Policy Formulation in Sweden," *Scandinavian Political Studies* 4: 103–16.

Meindl, R. S., and A. C. Swedlund. 1977. "Secular Trends in Mortality in the Connecticut Valley," *Human Biology* 49: 389–414.

Melosh, Barbara. 1982. *"The Physician's Hand": Work Culture and Conflict in American Nursing* (Philadelphia: Temple University Press).

Merton, Robert K. 1957. *Social Theory and Social Structure* (Glencoe, Ill.: Free Press).

Meyer, Jack A. 1981. "Health Care Competition: Are Tax Incentives Enough?" in

Mancur Olson, ed., *A New Approach to the Economics of Health Care* (Washington, D.C.: American Enterprise Institute for Public Policy Research). 424–49.

Meyer, John W., and Michael Hannan, eds. 1979. *National Development and the World System: Educational, Economic, and Political Change, 1950–1970* (Chicago: University of Chicago Press).

Meyer, John W., and Brian Rowan. 1977. "Institutionalized Organizations: Formal Structure as Myth and Ceremony," *American Journal of Sociology* 83.2: 340–63.

Meyer, John W., and W. Richard Scott. 1983. *Organizational Environments: Ritual and Rationality* (Beverly Hills, Calif.: Sage).

Meyer, John W., et al. 1979. "Public Education in the American States, 1870–1930," *American Journal of Sociology* 85: 591–613.

Meyer, Marshall. 1968a. "Automation and Bureaucratic Structure," *American Journal of Sociology* 74 (November): 256–64.

Meyer, Marshall. 1968b. "Expertness and the Span of Control," *American Sociological Review* 33 (December): 944–50.

Meyer, Marshall. 1968c. "Two Authority Structures of Bureaucratic Organizations," *Administrative Science Quarterly* 13 (September): 211–29.

Meyer, Marshall. 1972. "Size and the Structure of Organizations: A Causal Analysis," *American Sociological Review* 37 (August): 434–41.

Meyer, Marshall W., and M. Craig Brown. 1977. "Institutionalized Organizations: Formal Structures as Myth and Ceremony," *American Journal of Sociology* 83 (September): 340–63.

Michels, Robert. 1962. *Political Parties: A Sociological Study of the Oligarchical Tendencies of Modern Democracy* (New York: Collier Books).

Miller, S. M. 1987. "Race in the Health of America," *Milbank Quarterly* 65, Supplement 2: 500–31.

Ministère de la Santé et de la Sécurité Sociale. Various years. *Annuaire des statistiques sanitaires et sociales* (Paris: Ministère de la Santé et de la Sécurité Sociale).

Mintzberg, Henry. 1979. *The Structuring of Organizations* (Englewood Cliffs, N.J.: Prentice-Hall).

Mizrahi, A., and A. Mizrahi. 1979. *Quelques données Récentes sur la concentration des dépenses médicales* (Paris: Centre de Recherche pour L'Etude et L'Observation des Conditions de Vie, March).

Moch, Michael. 1976. "Structure in Organizational Resource Allocation," *Administrative Science Quarterly* 21 (December): 661–74.

Monsma, George N., Jr. 1970. "Marginal Revenue and the Demand for Physicians' Services," in Herbert E. Larman, ed., *Empirical Studies in Health Economics* (Baltimore: Johns Hopkins University Press), 145–60.

Musgrave, Richard A., and Peggy B. Musgrave. 1973. *Public Finance in Theory and Practice* (New York: McGraw-Hill).

Myers, George C., and Kenneth G. Manton. 1984. "Compression of Mortality: Myth or Reality," *Gerontologist* 24 (August): 346–59.

Mytinger, R. E. 1968. *Innovation in Local Health Services*, Public Health Service Publication no. 1664-2 (Washington, D. C.: GPO).

Narain, Francis, et al. 1976. *Evaluation Bibliometrics: The Use of Publications and Citations Analyses in the Evaluation of Scientific Activity* (Cherry Hill, N.J.: Computer Horizons).

National Center for Health Statistics. 1972. *Infant Mortality Rates: Socio-economic Factors*, ser. 22, no. 14 (Washington, D.C.: GPO).

National Center for Health Statistics, S. Sandier. 1983. "Comparison of Health Expenditures in France and the United States, 1950–1978," *Vital and Health Statistics*, ser. 3, no. 21 (Washington, D.C.: GPO).

Navarro, Vincente. 1976. "Social Class, Political Power, and the State and Their Implications in Medicine," *Social Science and Medicine* 10 (September/October): 437–57.

Navarro, Vincente. 1978a. *Class Struggle, the State, and Medicine: An Historical and Contemporary Analysis of the Medical Sector in Great Britain* (New York: Proclist).

Navarro, Vincente. 1978b. "The Crisis of the Western System of Medicine in Contemporary Capitalism," *International Journal of Health Services* 8: 179–211.

Navarro, Vincente. 1980. "Work, Ideology, and Science: The Case of Medicine," *International Journal of Health Services* 10: 523–50.

Navarro, Vincente. 1987. "Federal Health Policies in the United States: An Alternative Explanation," *Milbank Quarterly*, 65.1: 81–111.

Nerlove, Marc. 1971. "Further Evidence on the Estimation of Dynamic Economic Relations from a Time Series of Cross Sections," *Econometrica* 39: 359–82.

Newhouse, Joseph P. 1978. *The Economics of Medical Care* (Reading, Mass.: Addison-Wesley).

Newhouse, Joseph P., and Lindy J. Friedlander. 1980. "The Relationship between Medical Resources and Measures of Health: Some Additional Evidence," *Journal of Human Resources* 15 (Spring): 200–18.

New York Times. January 12, 1988. "Insurance Rates for Health Care Increase Sharply."

Noble, David F. 1977. *America by Design: Science, Technology, and the Rise of Corporate Capitalism* (New York: Alfred Knopf).

Noble, David F. 1984. *Forces of Production: A Social History of Industrial Automation* (New York: Alfred Knopf).

North, Douglass. 1981. *Structure and Change in Economic History* (New York: W. W. Norton).

Novak, S. J. 1973. "Professionalism and Bureaucracy: English Doctors and the Victorian Public Health Administration," *Journal of Social History* 6: 440–62.

Numbers, Ronald L. 1978. *Almost Persuaded: American Physicians and Compulsory Health Insurance, 1912–1920* (Baltimore: Johns Hopkins University Press).

O'Connor, James. 1973. *The Fiscal Crises of the State* (New York: St. Martin's Press).

Oddy, Derek J. 1970. "Working-Class Diets in Late Nineteenth-Century Britain," *Economic History Review*, 2d ser., 23 (August): 314–23.

Oddy, Derek J. 1982. "The Health of the People," in T. C. Barker and M. Drake, eds., *Population and Society in Britain, 1850–1980* (London: Batsford Academic and Educational), 121–39.

Oddy, Derek J. 1983. "Urban Famine in Nineteenth-Century Britain: The Effect of the Lancashire Cotton Famine on Working-Class Diet and Health," *Economic History Review* 36: 68–86.

Oddy, Derek J., and Derek S. Miller, eds. 1976. *The Making of the Modern British Diet* (London: Croom Helm).

Office of Health Economics. 1978. *Renal Failure: A Priority in Health?* (London: Office of Health Economics).

Office of Health Economics. 1980. *End-Stage Renal Failure* (London: Office of Health Economics).

Olson, Mancur. 1981. *A New Approach to the Economics of Health Care* (Washington, D.C.: American Enterprise Institute for Policy Research).

Organization for Economic Cooperation and Development. 1977. *Public Expenditure on Health*, OECD, Studies in Resource Allocation, no. 4 (Paris: OECD, July).

Organization for Economic Cooperation and Development. 1985. *Measuring Health Care, 1960–1983*. OECD Social Policy Studies, no. 2 (Paris: OECD).

Orloff, Ann S., and Theda Skocpol. 1984. "Why Not Equal Protection? Explaining the Politics of Public Social Spending in Britain, 1900–1911, and the United States, 1880s–1920," *American Sociological Review* 49 (December): 726–50.

Pamuk, Elsie R. 1985. "Social Class Inequality in Mortality from 1921 to 1972 in England and Wales," *Population Studies* 39: 17–31.

Parish, H. J. 1968. *Victory with Vaccines: The Story of Immunization* (Edinburgh: E. and S. Livingston).

Parker, Julia, et al. 1972. "Health," in A. H. Halsey, ed., *Trends in British Society since 1900* (London: Macmillan).

Paulston, R. G. 1968. *Swedish Comprehensive School Reform, 1918–1950: The Period of Formulation and Adoption* (New York: Columbia University Press).

Peabody, Susan Wade. 1909. "Historical Study of Legislation regarding Public Health in the States of New York and Massachusetts," *Journal of Infectious Diseases*, Supplement no. 4.

Peacock, Alan T., and Jack Wiseman. 1961. *The Growth of Public Expenditure in the United Kingdom* (Princeton: Princeton University Press).

Pedhazur, Elazer J. 1982. *Multiple Regression in Behavioral Research: Explanation and Prediction* (New York: Holt, Rinehart, and Winston).

Perlman, Mark, ed. 1974. *The Economics of Health and Medical Care* (New York: John Wiley).

Perrow, Charles. 1961a. "The Analysis of Goals in Complex Organizations," *American Sociological Review* 26 (December): 854–66.

Perrow, Charles. 1961b. "Organizational Prestige: Some Functions and Dysfunctions," *American Journal of Sociology* 66 (January): 335–41.

Perrow, Charles. 1967. "A Framework for the Comparative Analysis of Organizations," *American Sociological Review* 32 (April): 194–208.

Petersdorf, Robert G. 1985. "A Proposal for Financing Graduate Medical Education," *New England Journal of Medicine* 312 (May 16): 1322–24.

Peterson, A. D. C. 1952. *A Hundred Years of Education* (London: Duckworth).

Peterson, M. Jeanne. 1978. *The Medical Professional in Mid-Victorian London* (Berkeley: University of California Press).

Pfeffer, Jeffrey, and Gerald Salancik. 1978. *The External Control of Organizations: A Resource Dependence Perspective* (New York: Harper and Row, 1978).

Piore, Michael J., and Charles F. Sabel. 1984. *The Second Industrial Divide* (New York: Basic Books).

Political and Economic Planning. 1937. *Report on the British Health Services* (London: Political and Economic Planning).

Pooley, Marilyn E., and Colin G. Pooley. 1984. "Health, Society, and Environment in Nineteenth Century Manchester," in Robert Woods and John Woodward, eds., *Urban Disease and Mortality in Nineteenth Century England* (New York: St. Martin's Press), 148–75.

Powles, John. 1973. "On the Limitations of Modern Man," *Science, Medicine, and Man* 1 (April): 1–30.

Preston, Samuel H. 1976. *Mortality Patterns in National Populations: With Special Reference to Recorded Causes of Death* (New York: Academic Press).

Preston, Samuel H. 1977. "Mortality Trends," in Alex Inkeles, James Coleman, and Neil Smelser, eds., *Annual Review of Sociology* 3: 163–78.

Preston, Samuel H., and Etienne Van de Walle. 1978. "Urban French Mortality in the Nineteenth Century," *Population Studies* 32 (July): 275–97.

Price, Derek John de Solla. 1963. *Little Science, Big Science* (New York: Columbia University Press).

Price, James L. 1968. *Organizational Effectiveness: An Inventory of Propositions* (Homewood, Ill.: R. D. Irwin).

Prost, Antoine. 1988. *L'enseignement dans les pays du Marché Comun* (Paris: Armand Colin).

Prottas, Jeffrey, Mark Segal, and Harvey M. Sapolsky. 1983. "Cross-National Differences in Dialysis Rates," *Health Care Financing Review* 4 (March): 91–103.

Pryor, Frederick. 1968. *Public Expenditures in Communist and Capitalist Nations* (Homewood, Ill.: R. D. Irwin).

Quadagno, Jill S. 1984. "Welfare Capitalism and the Social Security Act of 1935," *American Sociological Review* 49 (October): 632–47.

Quadagno, Jill S. 1987. "Theories of the Welfare State," *Annual Review of Sociology* (Greenwich, Conn.: Jai Press), 151–74.

Rao, Potluri, and Roger LeRoy Miller. 1971. *Applied Econometrics* (Belmont, Calif.: Wadsworth).

Redfield, Robert, et al. 1936. "Memorandum on the Study of Acculturation," *American Anthropologist* 38 (January–March): 149–52.

Rein, Martin. 1969. "Social Class and the Utilization of Medical Care Services," *Hospitals* 43 (July 1): 43–54.

Reinhard, Uwe E. 1975. *Physician Productivity and the Demand for Health Manpower* (Cambridge, Mass.: Ballinger), 11.

Rettig, R. A. 1986. "The Policy Debate on Patient Care Financing for Victims of End-Stage Renal Disease," *Law and Contemporary Problems* 40: 196–230.

Rettig, R. A., and E. L. Marks. 1981. *Implementing the End-Stage Renal Disease Program of Medicare* (Washington, D.C.: U.S. Department of Health and Human Services).

Rice, Thomas. 1987. "An Economic Assessment of Health Care Coverage for the Elderly," *Milbank Quarterly* 65: 489–520.

Riley, James C. 1986. "Insects and the European Mortality Decline," *American Historical Review* 91 (October): 833–58.

Rinehart, Sue Tolleson. 1986. "Maternal Health Care Policy: Britain and the United States." Unpublished paper.

Ringer, Fritz. 1979. *Education and Society in Modern Europe* (Bloomington: Indiana University Press).

Robinson, Sail B., and J. Caspar Kuhlmann. 1967. "Two Decades of Non-reform in West German Education," *Comparative Education Review* 11 (October): 311–30.

Rochaix, Maurice. 1959. *Essai sur l'évolution des questions hospitalières de la fin de l'ancien régime a nos jours* (Paris: Fédération Hospitalière de France).

Rodwin, Victor G. 1982. "Management without Objectives: The French Health Policy Gamble," in Gordon McLachlan and Alan Maynard, eds., *The Public/Private Mix for Health: The Relevance and Effects of Change* (London: Nuffield Provincial Hospitals Trust), 289–321.

Rodwin, Victor G. 1984. *The Health Planning Predicament: France, Quebec, England, and the United States* (Berkeley: University of California Press).

Rogers, Everett M. 1962. *Diffusion of Innovations* (New York: Free Press).

Rösch, G., and Division d'Economie Médicale du Centre de Recherche pour l'Etude et l'Observation des Conditions de Vie. 1973. *Elements de "économique médicale"* (Paris: Flammarion).

Rösch, G., and S. Sandier. 1976. "A Comparison in the Health-Care Systems of France and the United States," in T. W. Hu, ed., *International Health Costs and Expenditures*, DHEW pub. no. (NIH) 76-1067, National Institutes of Health (Washington, D.C.: GPO).

Rosen, George. 1958. *A History of Public Health* (New York: M.D. Publications).

Rosen, George. 1964. "The Bacteriological, Immunologic, and Chemotherapeutic Period, 1875–1950," *Bulletin of the New York Academy of Medicine* 40 (June): 483–94.

Rosenberg, Charles E. 1962. *The Cholera Years: The United States in 1832, 1849, and 1866* (Chicago: University of Chicago Press).

Rosenberg, Charles E. 1977. "The Therapeutic Revolution: Medicine, Meaning, and Social Change in Nineteenth-Century America," *Perspectives in Biology and Medicine* 20: 485–516.

Rosenberg, Charles E. 1987. *The Care of Strangers: The Rise of America's Hospital System* (New York: Basic Books).

Rosenkrantz, Barbara. 1972. *Public Health and the State* (Cambridge: Harvard University Press).

Rosenthal, Marilynn M. 1986. "Beyond Equity: Swedish Health Policy and the Private Sector," *Milbank Quarterly* 64.4: 592–621.

Rosenwaike, Ira. 1985. "A Demographic Portrait of the Oldest Old," *Milbank Memorial Fund Quarterly* 63 (Spring): 187–205.

Rosenwaike, Ira, Yaffe Nurit, and Philip C. Sagi. 1980. "The Recent Decline in Mortality of the Extreme Aged: An Analysis of Statistical Data," *American Journal of Public Health* 70 (October): 1074–80.

Rosner, David A. 1982. *Once Charitable Enterprise: Hospitals and Health Care in Brooklyn and New York, 1885–1915* (Cambridge: Cambridge University Press).

Rostow, Dankwart. 1955. *The Politics of Compromise: A Study of Parties and Cabinet Government in Sweden* (Princeton: Princeton University Press).

Rothstein, William G. 1972. *American Physicians in the Nineteenth Century* (Baltimore: Johns Hopkins University Press).

Rowntree, B. Seebohm. 1908. *Poverty: A Study of Town Life* (London: Macmillan).

Russell, Louise B. 1977. "Diffusion of Hospital Technologies: Some Econometric Evidence," *Journal of Human Resources* 12 (Fall): 482–502.

Russell, Louise B. 1981. "An Aging Population and the Use of Medical Care," *Medical Care* 19 (June): 633–43.

Sabel, Charles F. 1982. *Work and Politics: The Division of Labor in Industry* (Cambridge: Cambridge University Press).

Saltman, Richard B. 1985. "The Capital Decision-Making Process in Regionalized Public Health Systems: Some Evidence from Sweden and Denmark," *Health Policy* 4: 279–89.

Santé et prestations sociales. 1971. Sixth National Economic Plan (Paris: Documentation Française).

Schlesinger, Mark, et al. 1987. "The Privatization of Health Care and Physicians' Perceptions to Hospital Services," *Milbank Quarterly* 65.1: 25–58.

Schmidt, William M. 1973. "The Development of Health Services for Mothers and Children in the United States," *American Journal of Public Health* 63 (May): 419–27.

Schmitter, Philippe. 1977. "Modes of Interest Intermediation and Models of Societal Change in Western Europe," *Comparative Political Studies* 10 (April): 7–38.

Schmockler, J. 1966. *Invention and Economic Growth* (Cambridge: Harvard University Press).

Schneyer, Solomon, J. Steven Landefield, and Frank H. Sandifer. 1981. "Bio-medical Research and Illness, 1900–1979," *Milbank Memorial Fund Quarterly* 59 (Winter): 44–58.

Schofield, R. 1983. "The Impact of Scarcity and Plenty on Population Change in England, 1541–1871," *Journal of Interdisciplinary History* 14: 265–91.

Schwartz, William B., et al. 1980. "The Changing Geographic Distribution of Board-Certified Physicians," *New England Journal of Medicine* 303 (October 30): 1032–38.

Schwartz, William B., et al. 1988. "Are We Training Too Many Medical Subspecialists?" *Journal of the American Medical Association* 259: 233–39.

Scott, W. Richard. 1982. "Health Care Organizations in the 1980s: The Convergence of the Public and Professional Control Systems," in Allen W. Johnson, et al., *Contemporary Health Services: Social Science Perspectives* (Boston: Auburn House).

Scott, W. Richard. 1987. "The Adolescence of Institutional Theory," *Administrative Science Quarterly* 32 (December): 493–511.

Seale, J. R. 1959. "A General Theory of National Expenditure on Medical Care," *Lancet* 2 (October 10): 555–59.

Sedgwick, W. T., and J. Scott MacNutt. 1910. "On the Mills-Reincke Phenomenon and Hazen's Theorem concerning the Decrease in Mortality from Diseases Other Than Typhoid Fever following the Purification of Public Water-Supplies," *Journal of Infectious Diseases* 7: 489–508.

Sempos, Christopher, et al. 1988. "Divergence of the Recent Trends in Coronary Mortality for the Four Major Race-Sex Groups in the United States," *American Journal of Public Health* 78 (November): 1422–27.

Serner, U. 1980. "Swedish Health Legislation: Milestones in Reorganization since 1945," in A. J. Heidenheimer and N. Elvander, eds., *The Shaping of the Swedish Health System* (New York: St. Martin's Press), 99–116.

Shah, Forida K., and Helen Abbey. 1971. "Effects of Some Factors on Neonatal and Postnatal Mortality," *Milbank Memorial Fund Quarterly* 49 (January): 33–57.

Shalev, Michael. 1983. "The Social Democratic Model and Beyond: Two Generations of Comparative Research on the Welfare State," *Comparative Social Research* 6: 87–148.

Shammas, Carole. 1983. "Food Expenditures and Economic Well-Being in Early Modern England," *Journal of Economic History* 43: 89–100.

Shammas, Carole. 1984. "The Eighteenth-Century English Diet and Economic Change," *Explorations in Economic History* 21: 254–69.

Shapiro, S., et al. 1980. "Relevance of Correlates of Infant Deaths for Significant Morbidity at 1 Year of Age," *American Journal of Obstetrics* 136: 363–73.

Shattuck, Lemuel. 1948. *Report of the Sanitary Commission of Massachusetts (1850)* (Cambridge: Harvard University Press).

Sheldon, Eleanor, and Wilbert Moore, eds. 1968. *Indicators of Social Change* (New York: Russell Sage Foundation).

Shepard, Herbert A. 1967. "Innovation-Resisting and Innovation-Producing Organizations," *Journal of Business* 40 (October): 470–77.

Sidel, Victor W., and Ruth Sidel. 1977. *A Healthy State: An International Perspective on the Crisis in United States Medical Care* (New York: Pantheon).

Simanis, J. G. 1973 "Medical Care Expenditures in Seven Countries," *Social Security Bulletin* 36 (March): 39–42.

Simon, John. 1857. "Papers Relating to the History and Practice of Vaccinations," *Parliamentary Papers, 1857 (2)*, vol. 35 (London: HMSO).

Skocpol, Theda. 1979. *States and Social Revolutions: A Comparative Analysis of France, Russia, and China* (Cambridge: Cambridge University Press).

Skocpol, Theda. 1981. "Political Response to Capitalist Crisis: Neo-Marxist Theories of the State and the Case of the New Deal," *Politics and Society* 2: 155–201.

Skocpol, Theda, and Edwin Amenta. 1986. "States and Social Policies," *Annual Review of Sociology* (Palo Alto, Calif.: Annual Reviews).

Skocpol, Theda, and John Ikenberry. 1983. "The Political Formation of the American Welfare State in Historical and Comparative Perspective," *Comparative Social Research* (Greenwich, Conn.: Jai Press).

Sloan, F. A., and R. Feldman. 1978. "Competition among Physicians," in W. Greenberg, ed., *Competition in the Health Care Sector*, Proceedings of a conference sponsored by the Bureau of Economics, Federal Trade Commission (Germantown, Md.: Aspen Systems).

Smillie, W. G. 1955. *Public Health: Its Promise for the Future* (New York: Macmillan).

Smith, F. B. 1979. *The People's Health, 1830–1910* (London: Croom Helm).

Sokoloff, K. L., and G. C. Villaflor. 1982. "The Early Achievement of Modern Stature in America," *Social Science History* 6: 453–81.

Spicer, C. C., and L. Lipworth. 1966. *Regional and Social Factors in Infant Mortality*, Studies on Medical and Population Subjects, no. 19 (London: HMSO).

Stamler, J. 1981. "Primary Prevention of Coronary Heart Disease: The Last Twenty Years," *American Journal of Cardiology* 47: 722–35.

Stamler, J. 1985. "Coronary Heart Disease: Doing the 'Right Things,'" *New England Journal of Medicine* 312: 1053–55.

Starr, Paul. 1982. *The Social Transformation of American Medicine* (New York: Basic Books).

Starr, Paul. 1985. "The Meaning of Privatization," *Working Paper No. 6: Privatization* (Washington, D.C.: National Conference on Social Welfare).

Steinwald, Bruce, and Frank A. Sloan. 1980. "Regulatory Approaches to Hospital Cost Containment: A Synthesis of Empirical Evidence" (Paper presented before the conference on health care sponsored by American Enterprise Institute for Public Policy Research, September).

Stephens, John D. 1979. *The Transition from Capitalism to Socialism* (New York: Macmillan).

Steudler, François. 1972. *Sociologie médicale*, coll. U2 (Paris: Armand Colin).

Steudler, François. 1973. "Le système hospitalier: Évolution et transformation" (Ph.D. diss., Centre d'Étude des Mouvements Sociaux, Paris).

Stevens, Rosemary. 1966. *Medical Practice in Modern England: The Impact of Specialization and State Medicine* (New Haven: Yale University Press).

Stevens, Rosemary. 1971. *American Medicine and the Public Interest* (New Haven: Yale University Press).

Stevens, Rosemary. 1989. *In Sickness and in Wealth: American Hospitals in the Twentieth Century* (New York: Basic Books).

Stewart, Charles T., Jr. 1971. "Allocation of Resources to Health," *Journal of Human Resources* 6 (Winter): 103–22.

Stone, Deborah A. 1984. *The Disabled State* (Philadelphia: Temple University Press).

Stone, Lawrence, ed. 1976. *Schooling and Society* (Baltimore: Johns Hopkins University Press).

Streeck, Wolfgang, and Philippe C. Schmitter. 1985. *Private Interest Government: Beyond Market and State* (Beverly Hills: Sage).

Taeuber, Conrad, and Irene B. Taeuber. 1958. *The Changing Population of the United States* (New York: John Wiley).

Tanner, J. M. 1978. *Fetus into Man: Physical Growth from Conception to Maturity* (Cambridge: Harvard University Press).

Tanner, J. M. 1981. *A History of the Study of Human Growth* (Cambridge: Cambridge University Press).

Tarr, Joel, James McCurley, and Terry F. Yosie. 1980. "The Development and Impact of Urban Wastewater Technology: Changing Concepts of Water Quality Control, 1850–1930." In Martin V. Melosi, ed., *Pollution and Reform in American Cities, 1870–1930* (Austin: University of Texas Press), 59–82.

Tarr, Joel, and Francis Clay McMichael, eds. 1977. *Retrospective Assessment of Wastewater Technology in the United States, 1800–1972* (Springfield, Va.: U.S. Department of Commerce, National Technical Information Service).

Temin, Peter. 1980. *Taking Your Medicine: Drug Regulation in the United States* (Cambridge: Harvard University Press).

Terris, Milton. 1980. "Epidemiology as a Guide to Health Policy," *Annual Review of Public Health* 1: 323–44.

Thomas, Lewis. 1977. "On the Science and Technology of Medicine," in John H. Knowles, ed., *Doing Better and Feeling Worse: Health in the United States* (New York: W. W. Norton), 35–46.

Thompson, Barbara. 1984. "Infant Mortality in Nineteenth-Century Bradford," in Robert Woods and John Woodward, eds., *Urban Disease and Mortality in Nineteenth-Century England* (New York: St. Martin's Press), 120–47.

Thompson, James D. 1967. *Organizations in Action* (New York: McGraw-Hill).

Thorsen, Laurence C. 1974. "How Can the U.S. Government Control Physician's Fees under National Health Insurance? A Lesson from the French System," *International Journal of Health Services* 4 (May): 49–57.

Tilly, Charles, ed. 1975. *The Formation of National States in Western Europe* (Princeton: Princeton University Press).

Tilton, Timothy. 1974. "The Social Origins of Liberal Democracy: The Swedish Case," *American Political Science Review* 68: 561–71.

Titmuss, Richard M. 1943. *Birth, Poverty, and Wealth* (London: Hamish Hamilton Medical Books).

Titmuss, Richard M. 1958. *Essays on the Welfare State* (Boston: Beacon Press).

Top, Franklin H., and Paul F. Wehrle. 1976. *Communicable and Infectious Diseases* (St. Louis, Mo.: C. V. Mosby).

Townsend, Peter, and Nick Davidson, eds. 1982. *Inequalities in Health: The Black Report* (Middlesex: Penguin Books).

Trussel, Ray, Mildred Morehead, and June Erlich. 1961. *The Quantity, Quality, and Costs of Medical and Hospital Care Secured by a Sample of Teamster Families in the New York Area* (New York: Columbia University School of Public Health).

Tuma, Nancy Brandon, and Michael T. Hannan. 1984. *Social Dynamics: Models and Methods* (Orlando, Fl.: Academic Press).

Twaddle, Andrew C., and Richard M. Hessler. 1986. "Power and Change: The Case of the Swedish Commission of Inquiry on Health and Sickness Care," *Journal of Health Politics, Policy, and Law* 11 (Spring): 19–40.

United Nations. 1954. *Foetal, Infant, and Early Childhood Mortality* (New York: United Nations).

United States Census Bureau. 1896. *Report on Vital and Social Statistics in the United States at the Eleventh Census*, pt. 1: *Analysis and Rate Tables* (Washington, D.C.: GPO).

United States Census Bureau. 1902. *1900 Census Reports*, vol. 3: *Vital Statistics*, pt. 1: *Analysis and Ratio Tables* (Washington, D.C.: U.S. Census Office), cclx, cclxi.

United States Census Bureau. 1979. *Vital Statistics of the United States, 1975* (Hyattsville, Md.: National Center for Health Statistics).

United States Census Bureau. Various years. *Vital Statistics of the United States* (Annual Reports) (Washington, D.C.: GPO).

United States Congress, Office of Technology Assessment. 1981. *Patent-Term Extension and the Pharmaceutical Industry* (Washington, D.C.: GPO).

United States Department of Health and Human Services. 1983. "Comparison of Health Expenditures in France and the United States, 1950–1978," *Analytical and Epidemiological Studies*, ser. 3 (Hyattsville, Md.: National Center for Health Statistics).

United States House of Representatives. 1988. *Hearings on Equal Access to Health Care: Patient Dumping*, Committee on Government Operations, 100th cong.

United States Senate. 1973. *Hearings on Competitive Problems in the Drug Industry*, Subcommittee on Monopoly of Select Committee on Small Business, 93d cong.

Vinovskis, M. A. 1972. "Mortality Rates and Trends in Massachusetts before 1860," *Journal of Economic History* 32: 184–213.

Vogel, Morris. 1980. *The Invention of the Modern Hospital: Boston, 1870–1930* (Chicago: University of Chicago Press).

Waaler, H. Th. 1984. *Height, Weight, and Mortality: The Norwegian Experience*, Gruppe for Helsetjenesteforskning, report no. 4, Oslo.

Wagner, Adolph. 1958. "Three Extracts on Public Finance," in Richard A. Musgrave and Alan Peacock, eds., *Classics in the Theory of Public Finance* (New York: Macmillan), 1–16.

Waldron, H. A., and I. Vickerstaff. 1977. *Intimations of Quality: Ante-Mortem and Post-Mortem Diagnoses* (London: Nuffield Provincial Hospitals Trust).

Walker, Jack L. 1971. "Innovation in State Politics," in Herbert Jacobs and Kenneth Vines, eds., *Politics in the American States: A Comparative Analysis* (Boston: Little, Brown).

Wallace, T. D., and Ashiq Hussain. 1969. "The Use of Error Components Models in Combining Cross-Section with Time-Series Data," *Econometrica* 37: 55–67.

Walters, Pamela B., and Richard Rubinson. 1983. "Educational Expansion and Economic Output in the United States," *American Sociological Review* 48: 480–93.

Ward, Richard A. 1975. *The Economics of Health Resources* (Reading, Mass.: Addison-Wesley).

Ward, W. Peter, and Patricia C. Ward. 1984. "Infant Birth Weight and Nutrition in Industrializing Montreal," *American Historical Review* 89: 324–45.

Wardell, William. 1973a. "British and American Awareness of Some New Therapeutic Drugs," *Clinical Pharmacology and Therapeutics* 14 (November–December): 1022–34.

Wardell, William. 1973b. "Introduction to New Therapeutic Drugs in the United States and Great Britain: An International Comparison," *Clinical Pharmacology and Therapeutics* 14 (September–October): 773–90.

Wardell, William. 1975. "Developments in the Introduction of New Drugs in the United States and Britain, 1971–1974," in Robert B. Helms, ed., *Drug Development and Marketing* (Washington, D.C.: American Enterprise Institute for Public Policy), 165–81.

Wardell, William M., and Louis Lasagna. 1975. *Regulation and Drug Development* (Washington, D.C.: American Enterprise Institute).

Weber, Max. 1947. *The Theory of Social and Economic Organization*, trans. A. M. Henderson and Talcott Parsons (New York: Free Press of Glencoe).

Weber, Max. 1958. *From Max Weber: Essays in Sociology*, trans. Hans Gerth and C. W. Mills (New York: Oxford University Press).

Weber, Max. 1968. *Economy and Society*, trans. Guenther Roth and Claus Wittich (New York: Bedminister Press).

Weher, Phillip G. 1987. "The Public Health Impact of Alzheimer's Disease," *American Journal of Public Health* 77: 1157–58.

Weisbrod, Burton A. 1977. *The Voluntary Nonprofit Sector* (Lexington, Mass.: Lexington Books).

Weisbrod, Burton A. 1988. *The Nonprofit Economy* (Cambridge: Harvard University Press).

Weller, Geoffrey R., and Pranial Manga. 1983. "The Push for Reprivatization of Health Care Services in Canada, Britain, and the United States," *Journal of Health Politics, Policy, and Law* (Fall): 495–518.

Whittet, T. D. 1970. "Drug Control in Britain: From World War I to the Medicines Act of 1968," in John B. Blake, ed., *Safeguarding the Public: Historical Aspects of Medicinal Drug Control* (Baltimore: Johns Hopkins University Press), 27–37.

Wilensky, Harold L. 1975. *The Welfare State and Equality* (Berkeley: University of California Press).

Wilensky, Harold L. 1976. *The "New Corporatism," Centralization, and the Welfare State* (Beverly Hills, Calif.: Sage).

Wilensky, Harold L., et al. 1985. *Comparative Social Policy: Theories, Methods, Findings* (Berkeley, Calif.: Institute of International Studies).

Wilensky, Harold, and Charles Lebeaux. 1965. *Industrial Society and Social Welfare*, enlarged paperback ed. (New York: Free Press).

Williams, Alan. 1978. "Efficiency and Welfare." In Sir Douglas Black and G. P. Thomas, eds., *Providing for the Health Services* (London: Croom Helm).

Williamson, J. G. 1976. "American Prices and Urban Inequality since 1820," *Journal of Economic History* 36: 303–33.

Williamson, J. G. 1981a. "Urban Disamenities, Dark Satanic Mills, and the British Standard of Living Debate," *Journal of Economic History* 41: 75–83.

Williamson, J. G. 1981b. "Some Myths Die Hard—Urban Disamenities One More Time: A Reply," *Journal of Economic History* 41: 905–7.

Williamson, J. G. 1982. "Was the Industrial Revolution Worth It? Disamenities and

Death in Nineteenth Century British Towns," *Explorations in Economic History* 19: 221–45.

Williamson, J. G., and P. H. Lindert. 1980. *American Inequality: A Microeconomic History* (New York: Academic Press).

Williamson, Oliver E. 1975. *Markets and Hierarchies—Analyses and Antitrust Implications: A Study in the Economics of International Organization* (New York: Free Press).

Williamson, Oliver E. 1981. "The Economics of Organization: The Transaction Cost Approach," *American Journal of Sociology* 87: 548–77.

Williamson, Oliver E. 1985. *The Economic Institutions of Capitalism* (New York: Free Press).

Willoughby, Gertrude. 1966. "Doctors and Patients in France," *New Society* 8 (December 22): 941–42.

Winich, M., and J. A. Brasel. 1980. "Nutrition and Cell Growth," in R. S. Goodhart and M. E. Shils, eds., *Nutrition in Health and Disease* (Philadelphia: Lea and Febiger), 592–607.

Winslow, C. E. A. 1923. *The Evolution and Significance of the Modern Public Health Campaign* (New Haven: Yale University Press).

Winslow, C. E. A. 1929. *The Life of Hermann M. Biggs* (Philadelphia: Lea and Febiger).

Winter, J. M. 1977. "The Impact of the First World War on Civilian Health in Britain," *Economic History Review*, 2d ser., 30: 487–507.

Wohl, Anthony. 1983. *Endangered Lives: Public Health in Victorian Britain* (London: Methuen).

Wonnacott, Ronald J., and Thomas H. Wonnacott. 1970. *Econometrics* (New York: John Wiley).

Woodbury, Robert M. 1925. *Causal Factors in Infant Mortality*, U.S. Children's Bureau Publication, no. 142, U.S. Labor Department (Washington, D.C.: GPO).

Woods, Robert. 1984. "Mortality Patterns in the Nineteenth Century," in Woods and John Woodward, eds., *Urban Disease and Mortality in Nineteenth-Century England* (New York: St. Martin's Press), 37–64.

Woods, Robert, and John Woodward, eds. 1984. *Urban Disease and Mortality in Nineteenth-Century England* (New York: St. Martin's Press, 1984).

Woodward, John. 1974. *Do the Sick No Harm* (London: Routledge and Kegan Paul).

Woodward, John. 1984. "Medicine and the City: Nineteenth-Century Experience," in Robert Woods and Woodward, eds., *Urban Disease and Mortality in Nineteenth-Century England* (New York: St. Martin's Press), 64–78.

Woodward, John, and David Richards, eds. 1977. *Health Care and Popular Medicine in Nineteenth-Century England: Essays in the Social History of Medicine* (London: Croom Helm).

Wrigley, E. A., and R. S. Schofield, 1981. *The Population History of England, 1541–1871: A Reconstruction* (London: Edward Arnold).

Yaggy, Duncan, ed. 1984. *Health Care for the Poor and Elderly* (Durham, N.C.: Duke University Press).

Yasuba, Yasukichi. 1962. *Birth Rates of the White Population in the United States, 1780–1860: An Economic Study* (Baltimore: Johns Hopkins University Press).

Youmans, Guy P., Philip Y. Patterson, and Herbert M. Sommers. 1975. *The Biological and Clinical Basis of Infectious Diseases* (Philadelphia: W. B. Saunders).

Zaltman, Gerald, Robert Duncan, and Jonny Holbek. 1973. *Innovations and Organizations* (New York: John Wiley).

Zey-Ferrell, Mary. 1979. *Dimensions of Organizations: Environment, Context, Structure, Process, and Performance* (Santa Monica, Calif.: Goodyear).

Zucker, Lynne G. 1983. "Organizations as Institutions," in S. B. Bacharach, ed., *Advances in Organizational Theory and Research* (Greenwich, Conn.: Jai Press).

Zucker, Lynne G. 1987. "Institutional Theories of Organization," *Annual Review of Sociology* 13: 443–64.

INDEX

Library of Congress Cataloging-in-Publication Data

Hollingsworth, J. Rogers (Joseph Rogers), 1932–
    State intervention in medical care : consequences, for Britain,
France, Sweden, and the United States, 1890–1970 / J. Rogers Hollingsworth,
Jerald Hage, and Robert Hanneman.
        p.   cm.
    Includes bibliographical references.
    ISBN 0-8014-2389-9 (alk. paper).
    ISBN 0-8014-9615-2 (pbk. alk. paper)
    1. Social medicine—Europe.   2. Social medicine—United States.
3. Medical policy—Europe.   4. Medical policy—United States.
I. Hage, Jerald, 1932–   .   II. Hanneman, Robert.   III. Title.
RA418.3.E85H65   1990
362.1'094—dc20   89-25155